Guidelines
for Graded Exercise Testing
and Exercise Prescription

Guidelines
for
Graded Exercise Testing
and
Exercise Prescription

AMERICAN COLLEGE OF SPORTS MEDICINE

Lea & Febiger · *Philadelphia*

Library of Congress Cataloging in Publication Data

American College of Sports Medicine.
    Guidelines for graded exercise testing and exercise pre-
scription.

    Includes index.
    1. Gymnastics, Medical. 2. Cardiovascular patient—Re-
habilitation. 3. Exercise tests. I. Title. [DNLM: 1. Exercise
test. 2. Exertion. 3. Exercise therapy. WE103 A514g]
RC684.E9A45 1975   615'.824   75-5894

ISBN   0-8121-0524-9

Reprinted, 1976

Published in Great Britain by Henry Kimpton Publishers,
London

PRINTED IN THE UNITED STATES OF AMERICA

Preface

The impetus for the American College of Sports Medicine to undertake the writing and publication of the Guidelines originated at a special interest group meeting on Cardiac Rehabilitation at the Annual Meeting of the American College of Sports Medicine held in Philadelphia on May 2, 1972. The recommendation from this meeting was that the American College of Sports Medicine should initiate some type of program to assist the many new groups who were starting exercise programs. A special Sub-Committee was formed by the Post-Graduate Education Committee to investigate the problem, set guidelines for possible American College of Sports Medicine Programs, and make recommendations for implementation. The six members of the Sub-Committee met in Washington in September, 1972. The Sub-Committee decided to develop guidelines for graded exercise testing and exercise prescription for both the healthy and the unhealthy, and behavioral objectives for the four key figures in the administration of graded exercise testing and conditioning programs: the physician, the program director, the exercise leader, and the exercise technician.

Sub-Committee members undertook specific writing assignments to prepare a working document for presentation at a workshop at Aspen, Colorado, in December, 1972. Fifteen laboratories actively engaged in graded exercise testing and exercise prescription were arbitrarily chosen and two members from each group were invited to participate. Eighteen people accepted and attended the 4-day workshop. Six small Discussion Groups worked on specific parts of the Guidelines or Behavioral Objectives and reported back to the total group for consensus.

Participants in the workshop undertook specific writing assignments and review tasks and a draft of the manuscript was compiled by February, 1973. The Sub-Committee reported the progress on the Guidelines and future plans for implementation at an open meeting during the 1973 Annual Meeting of the College at Seattle in May. The Sub-Committee had completed its task and was disbanded and the Post-Graduate Education Committee undertook to edit the manuscript throughout the summer and early fall. A final draft was typed and this served as a working document at an open workshop held at Aspen, Colorado, in December, 1973, attended by 55 persons from 32 laboratories. The objective was to give the document wider exposure prior to publication. Six sub-groups worked on exercise risk, screening and supervision, drugs and emergency procedures, sub-maximum compared to maximum tests, intensity and duration of exercise, and metabolic cost of physical activities. The revisions proposed by the sub-groups were presented to the total group for discussion. Sub-group chairmen then turned their final drafts over to the Publications Committee for final editing and publication.

The involvement of physicians, physiologists, and physical educators from 32 laboratories located in 19 different states and 3 Canadian provinces assures that the Guidelines reflect the many different views of graded exercise testing and exercise prescription. The format of the Guidelines was developed as a largely descriptive treatment of how to organize and administer graded exercise testing and prescription. No references were to be included in the text and since so many persons contributed no individual credits were to be made. The Guidelines include the application of testing and prescription procedures to the entire population. We realize that this is an ambitious undertaking but the diversity of the input from multidisciplinary groups who are currently administering programs assures us of a reasonable approach in terms of the current trends. The Behavioral Objectives are the first attempt to develop outlines of the competencies required for the personnel involved in exercise programs. The Behavioral Objectives should aid in the development of programs to prepare personnel for these programs and in the self-evaluation of workers in the field. The American College of Sports Medicine thanks the many workers who have contributed directly and indirectly to the development of these Guidelines and hopes that they provide a useful document for workers in the field of graded exercise testing and exercise prescription.

Contents

Appendix

Introduction

The proliferation in the number and types of adult exercise programs being conducted during the past few years has increased the need to establish guidelines for the safe and effective operation of these programs. The statement made by the American Heart Association's Committee on Exercise emphasized both the risks in exercise and the roles of exercise testing and exercise prescription.

> "For the sedentary individual there is serious risk in the sudden, unregulated and injudicious use of strenuous exercise. But it is a risk that can be minimized and perhaps even eliminated through proper preliminary testing and the individualized prescribing of exercise programs."

Unfortunately, the precise nature and magnitude of "risks"* cannot be estimated in definite terms of exercise

---

* To clarify the term "risk" used throughout these Guidelines the following definitions are suggested:
1. People "at risk" or "at high risk" are those who have a few, a majority, or all of the established risk factors pointing toward the potential development of coronary heart disease. An exercise testing and conditioning program is not necessarily dangerous to these people.
2. If used freely, the term "risk" or "high risk" is synonymous with "hazard," indicating an existing potential danger of unhealthy occurrences when individuals are physically stressed.

intensity and duration unless the functional capacity of the individual has been evaluated.

Exercise may have a place in the PREVENTION of atherosclerotic cardiovascular disease if it is proven that it reduces certain risk factors or has an independent beneficial effect. In REHABILITATION, the role of exercise in certain types of cardiovascular disease is established. As yet, there is inconclusive evidence that physically active people enjoy greater longevity or that they have a lower incidence of coronary heart disease than physically inactive people. In many of the studies reported the demonstrated differences were subject to bias by the self-selection of persons into active and inactive groups. Our knowledge is also limited because exercise cardiology and exercise prescription are relatively new study areas.

The current Guidelines for Exercise Testing and Exercise Prescription, which are assumed to be equally valid for both sexes and the entire age range, reflect an initial attempt to synthesize available knowledge into a workable format. Periodic revisions will be necessary as our knowledge and understanding of this complex area evolve.

The American College of Sports Medicine recognizes that there has been, and continues to be, a cultural trend toward physical inactivity for most residents of industrialized nations. This is of profound concern to the members of this and numerous other professional organizations and health agencies. Therefore, although not necessarily supported by definitive studies, the American College of Sports Medicine tentatively issues these policy statements.

1. When properly prescribed, physical activity is beneficial since it maintains or increases functional capacity and may modify some risk factors associated with atherosclerotic disease.
2. Physical activity, particularly when "sudden, unregulated and strenuous," constitutes a serious hazard to *some* persons.
3. With our present knowledge, most high risk individuals can be recognized by a proper medical examination *and* an appropriate graded exercise test.
4. Initial prescription and subsequent modifications can be safely determined from knowledge generated from repeated graded exercise tests.
5. The attainment and maintenance of functional capacity are an individual responsibility. However, the safe attainment of this is a concern of health and exercise professionals, particularly for those individuals considered "at risk" from an injudicious increase in their physical activity level.
6. In advance of or concomitant with large scale education and motivational endeavors to increase individual physical activity levels, it is desirable to identify and select that segment of the population "at risk." This would enable these individuals to benefit from suitable evaluation and a scientific application of controlled activity programming through exercise testing and exercise prescription. The remainder of the population could avail themselves of these same techniques for a variety of elective reasons.

7. The benefits of graded exercise testing and exercise prescription can only be realized when the physician, program director, exercise leader, and exercise technician have been well-trained and are competent in the roles they assume in the exercise program.

8. Exercise testing and exercise prescription, to be conducted most effectively and efficiently, require a multidisciplinary approach. This can be realized optimally with cooperative teamwork, a delegation and acceptance of responsibility, and adequate education to assure that personnel are well-trained and competent in the roles they assume in the exercise program.

9. Physicians involved in graded exercise testing and physical activity prescription in group programs, whether salaried, fee-for-service, or voluntary, in many instances are acting as consultants and are subject to the ethical considerations relating to consultants. Frequently, they do not and should not engage in the delivery of primary medical care to the patients in the program except as specifically requested by the patient's referring physician.

10. The American College of Sports Medicine is committed to providing assistance in the promulgation of these Guidelines and in the development of educational and liaison assistance toward the implementation of high quality exercise testing and prescribing programs in the United States and Canada.

Guidelines
for Admitting Adults
into Exercise Programs

Persons of any age may volitionally make significant increases in their habitual levels of physical activity without reference to either their personal physician or any organized program. If there are no contraindications to exercise and if a rational program is developed, the transition to a higher exercise level may be made satisfactorily. For the sedentary adult there is no assurance that there are not contraindications and that he can exercise safely. There is even less assurance that he will undertake exercises of the appropriate type, duration, intensity and frequency. Initially, sedentary adults should be encouraged to participate in a supervised program primarily to learn how to exercise properly. For high risk patients or those with known cardiovascular and/or pulmonary disease, any major increase in physical activity for the purposes of physical conditioning should be carried out under supervision. The following are the guidelines for the admission of adults into exercise programs.

PRELIMINARY MEDICAL EVALUATION

The major determinants in setting appropriate screening and supervisory procedures for graded exercise testing and exercise programs are the age and health status of the proposed participant. In order to recommend set procedures it is necessary to make some arbitrary separations in variables such as age, symptomatology and risk factors (Table 1). One might argue for either a

TABLE 1. CLASSIFICATION BY AGE AND HEALTH STATUS OF PARTICIPANTS WHO REQUIRE DIFFERENT SCREENING AND SUPERVISORY PROCEDURES DURING GRADED EXERCISE TESTING.

Age	*Health Status*
A. Less than 35 years	A. Asymptomatic
	1. No known risk factors
B. 35 years or older	2. Secondary risk factors
	3. Primary risk factors
	4. Documented coronary artery disease
	B. Symptomatic
	1. Suspected coronary artery disease
	2. Documented coronary artery disease

NOTE: Primary risk factors are hypertension, hyperlipidemia and cigarette smoking. Secondary risk factors are family history, obesity, physical inactivity, diabetes mellitus and asymptomatic hyperglycemia. The participant's status in the last two risk factors need not be determined in young (less than 35 years) asymptomatic participants with no risk factors. In participants 35 years of age or over, and in participants with risk factors or symptoms, blood lipids and blood glucose levels should be measured.

higher or lower separation age than 35 years and that smoking and sedentary living may well constitute primary risk factors. The age of 35 and the designations of health status are set on purely pragmatic grounds based upon the evaluation of many thousands of presumed normal individuals and patients with coronary heart disease (CHD).

A. Asymptomatic Individuals Under Age 35

For asymptomatic individuals less than 35 years of age, who have no previous history of cardiovascular disease or are not *known* to have any primary CHD risk factors, the risk of an increase in habitual physical activity is usually sufficiently low for them to proceed without any special medical clearance. However, if they have any questions about their health status, develop symptoms or have not had a medical examination during the past 2 years, they should consult with their personal physician. If the individual is less than 35 years of age and has no known primary CHD risk factors or symptoms, it is considered acceptable for him to perform a graded exercise test (for the purpose of preparing an exercise prescription) that may be administered by a trained exercise technician with no physician present during the test.

B. High Risk or Symptomatic Individuals and Those 35 Years of Age and Older

For individuals 35 or less with a history or any evidence of cardiovascular disease or with significant combinations of CHD risk factors including family history, elevated blood pressure, hyperlipidemia, diabetes, cigarette smoking or obesity, it is recommended that a medical evaluation be obtained prior to any major increase in physical activity. Regardless of health status, it is advisable that any adult above 35 years have a medical evaluation prior to a major increase in his exercise habits. It seems advisable that before any major increase in physical activity, persons above the age of 35 years or those who are under 35 and are either at high risk or are symptomatic take an ECG monitored exercise test under the supervision of a physician. If the participant is over 35 years of age or with participants of any age if the interview or examination uncovers major risk factors or symptoms, it seems advisable that an exercise test be conducted according to one of the following two protocols: 1) if the participant is 35 years of age or older or regardless of age has major risk factors or documented CHD but is asymptomatic, the graded exercise test may be administered by an exercise technician but a physician must be available in the test area. The physician must know that the graded exercise test is in progress, be responsible for the safety of the participant but not necessarily be in visual contact with the participant; and 2) if the participant regardless of age is symptomatic with either suspected or documented CHD, the graded exercise test may be administered by a physician or by an exercise technician but the physician must be in visual contact with the subject as he performs the test.

In summary, the current limited availability of qualified health personnel and facilities in relation to the large volume of medical evaluations and graded exercise testing required to comply with these recommendations necessitates a great deal of discretion in their implementation. Three protocols for supervision of graded exercise tests are proposed: 1) no physician present, 2) physician present but not in visual contact, and 3) physician in visual contact with the subject. The appropriate protocol is based on the age, magnitude of CHD risk factors, and symptomatology of the person to be tested.

Some physicians may find screening their patients prior to an increase in habitual exercise of great value in developing and maintaining rapport with their patients. These physicians may wish to handle screening as part of their private practice. Other physicians, because of a lack of facilities and/or trained personnel, will experience difficulty with exercise screening and exercise prescription. Under these circumstances, communities may wish to set up a central referral agency for the purpose of exercise testing, prescription and program supervision.

C. Medical Evaluation

The medical evaluation should elicit information that will aid the physician in making a decision regarding the plans of his patient to increase his physical activity. This includes:

1. Comprehensive medical history questionnaire or review. Family health history, personal medical history and current health related habits (*e.g.* cigarette smoking, diet, alcohol intake, habitual physical activity, medications, etc.). Special emphasis should be directed toward any history of chest pain, dysrhythmias, intermittent

TABLE 2. CONTRAINDICATIONS TO EXERCISE AND EXERCISE TESTING

I. Absolute Contraindications

1. Manifest circulatory insufficiency ("congestive heart failure")
2. Acute myocardial infarction
3. Active myocarditis
4. Rapidly increasing angina pectoris with effort
5. Recent embolism, either systemic or pulmonary
6. Dissecting aneurysm
7. Acute infectious disease
8. Thrombophlebitis
9. Ventricular tachycardia and other dangerous dysrhythmias (multifocal ventricular activity)
10. Severe aortic stenosis

II. Relative Contraindications*

1. Uncontrolled or high-rate supraventricular dysrhythmia
2. Repetitive or frequent ventricular ectopic activity
3. Untreated severe systematic or pulmonary hypertension
4. Ventricular aneurysm
5. Moderate aortic stenosis
6. Uncontrolled metabolic disease (diabetes, thyrotoxicosis, myxedema)
7. Severe myocardial obstructive syndromes (subaortic stenosis)
8. Marked cardiac enlargement
9. Toxemia of pregnancy

* In the practice of medicine the value of testing often exceeds the risk for patients with these relative contraindications.

TABLE 2. CONTRAINDICATIONS TO EXERCISE AND EXERCISE TESTING (Continued)

III. Conditions Requiring Special Consideration and/or Precautions

1. Conduction disturbance
   a) Complete atrioventricular block
   b) Left bundle branch block
   c) Wolff-Parkinson-White syndrome
2. Fixed rate pacemaker
3. Controlled dysrhythmia
4. Electrolyte disturbance
5. Certain medication
   a) Digitalis
   b) β-Blocking and drugs of related action

6. Clinically severe hypertension (diastolic over 110, grade III retinopathy)
7. Angina pectoris and other manifestations of coronary insufficiency
8. Cyanotic heart disease
9. Intermittent or fixed right-to-left shunt
10. Severe anemia
11. Marked obesity
12. Renal, hepatic and other metabolic insufficiency
13. Overt psychoneurotic disturbance requiring therapy
14. Neuromuscular, musculoskeletal or arthritic disorders which would prevent activity

claudication or other forms of cardiovascular disease. This history may be self-administered or conducted by an interviewer.

2. Physical examination. Emphasis on identifying symptoms and signs indicative of cardiopulmonary dis-

ease and other health problems that would be contra-indications to exercise testing (Table 2). The examination should include investigation of bone and joint abnormalities, cardiac murmurs and gallop sound, dysrhythmias, presence of chronic lung disease, edema, ascites, and xanthoma.

3. Twelve-lead resting electrocardiogram (ECG).

4. Resting systolic and diastolic blood pressure.

5. Blood analyses. Fasting blood glucose, cholesterol and triglyceride concentrations are recommended but not essential.

6. A graded, ECG monitored exercise test (unless medically contraindicated). Data collected during a graded exercise test may 1) be used to determine the physical work capacity in kgm/min or the functional capacity in METS (work metabolic rate/resting metabolic rate) of a subject; 2) serve as the basis for exercise prescription; 3) in conjunction with the medical history, physical examination, chest x-ray film, 12 lead resting ECG, and catheterization data, aid in the evaluation of cardiovascular disorders; or 4) assist in the selection and evaluation of appropriate modes of treatment.

Guidelines for Graded Exercise Test Administration

1. Contraindications to or Special Precautions During Exercise Testing. There are various contraindications to increased physical activity, whether it occurs as a result of a graded exercise test, occupational tasks, hobbies or sports. There are also conditions which might arise with each type of exercise test that require special precautions. These contraindications and precautions are listed in Table 2.

2. Informed Consent. The testing procedures must be carefully explained to the participant by either the attending physician or by the exercise technician. In particular, the participant must know exactly what is expected of him. Following the explanation of the test protocol, the participant must be asked if he has any questions and all questions must be answered fully. Then, if he is willing to take the test, the participant must sign the informed consent form (Appendix A).

3. Termination of Graded Exercise Test. When an exercise test is being conducted by a non-physician, it should be stopped for the following reasons. If a physician is conducting the test, he may decide to use other criteria.

   a. Symptoms of significant exertional intolerance.

      1. Dizziness or near syncope.

    2. Angina.

    3. Unusual or intolerable fatigue.

    4. Intolerable claudication or pain.

  b. Signs of intolerance.

    1. Staggering or unsteadiness.

    2. Mental confusion.

    3. Facial expression signifying disorders (strained or blank facies).

    4. Cyanosis or pallor (facial or elsewhere).

    5. Rapid distressful breathing.

    6. Nausea or vomiting.

    7. A definite fall in systolic blood pressure with increasing work load.

  c. Electrocardiographic changes.

    1. S–T segment displacement of 0.2 mV below the baseline.

    2. Supraventricular or ventricular dysrhythmias or ectopic ventricular activity occurring before the end of a T-wave (R-on-T phenomenon). It is recommended that a test be terminated in the presence of three or more successive ectopic ventricular complexes or with a significant increase in their occurrence (about 10 per minute depending on clinical judgment).

    3. Major left intraventricular conduction disturbances.

  d. Blood pressure responses.

Systolic blood pressure can be measured with reasonable accuracy by the auscultatory method during graded exercise on the bicycle ergometer or treadmill and with more difficulty with step climbing. An exercise test should be terminated if systolic blood pressure shows a definite decrease when the work load is further increased. No strict rule can be made as to the level of blood pressure at which the test should be terminated. In general, any increase in exercise intensity should be accompanied by an increase in systolic pressure. A distinct irreversible decline of the systolic blood pressure usually indicates significant cardiac dysfunction and serves as a useful criterion for test termination.

During graded exercise, measurement of the diastolic blood pressure by the auscultatory method is also of value in providing information relative to test termination: a rise in diastolic pressure of more than 20 mm Hg or a rise above 100 mm Hg is cause for concern and under most circumstances the test should be stopped.

    e. Heart rate responses.

The heart rate responses of persons are quite variable at rest, in anticipation of exercise, and during exercise. The variability is increased even further by age, physical conditioning and disease. The maximum heart rates of young college athletes may vary from 165 to 215 beats/min. Patients may have heart rates in maximum work of no higher than 80 beats/min. Gross estimates of maximum heart rates for different age groups are given in Table 3, but it is impossible to set useful maximum heart rates for specific individuals. Therefore, the termination of an exercise test on the basis of reaching 85 to 90% of a predicted maximum heart rate is of questionable validity. Once the maximum heart rate has been experimentally determined in a graded exercise test, it may be used effectively in exercise prescription.

TABLE 3. AVERAGE MAXIMUM HEART RATES BY AGE AND RECOMMENDED TARGET HEART RATES FOR NORMAL ASYMPTOMATIC PARTICIPANTS DURING EXERCISE.

Age by decade	20–29	30–39	40–49	50–59	60–69
Maximum heart rate	190	185	180	170	160
Peak .9(max HR−75)+75	179	174	170	161	152
Average .7(max HR−75) +75	155	152	149	141	135

NOTE: These are only approximations. Maximum heart rate varies greatly and should be determined for each subject. The maximum heart rates for patients may be much lower than these rates. For the calculations of the target heart rate, a resting heart rate of 75 beats/min was assumed.

4. The participant should have a recent standard 12-lead resting ECG before the exercise test (Appendix B).

5. Energy requirements during graded exercise are most readily communicated in METS. One MET is the equivalent of a resting oxygen consumption which is approximately 3.5 ml/kg min. METS during exercise are determined by dividing work metabolic rate by resting metabolic rate. The MET cost of treadmill work is independent of body weight, but the MET cost of bicycle ergometry is dependent on body weight (Table 4).

TABLE 4. ENERGY EXPENDITURE IN METS DURING BICYCLE ERGOMETRY.

Body Weight		Work Rate on Bicycle Ergometer (kg m⁻¹ min⁻¹ and Watts)												
(kg)	(lb)	75	150	300	450	600	750	900	1050	1200	1350	1500	1650	1800 (kg m⁻¹ min⁻¹)
		12	25	50	75	100	125	150	175	200	225	250	275	300 (Watts)
20	44	4.0	6.0	10.0	14.0	18.0	22.0							
30	66	3.4	4.7	7.3	10.0	12.7	15.3	17.9	20.7	23.3				
40	88	3.0	4.0	6.0	8.0	10.0	12.0	14.0	16.0	18.0	20.0	22.0		
50	110	2.8	3.6	5.2	6.8	8.4	10.0	11.5	13.2	14.8	16.3	18.0	19.6	21.1
60	132	2.7	3.3	4.7	6.0	7.3	8.7	10.0	11.3	12.7	14.0	15.3	16.7	18.0
70	154	2.6	3.1	4.3	5.4	6.6	7.7	8.8	10.0	11.1	12.2	13.4	14.0	15.7
80	176	2.5	3.0	4.0	5.0	6.0	7.0	8.0	9.0	10.0	11.0	12.0	13.0	14.0
90	198	2.4	2.9	3.8	4.7	5.6	6.4	7.3	8.2	9.1	10.0	10.9	11.8	12.6
100	220	2.4	2.8	3.6	4.4	5.2	6.0	6.8	7.6	8.4	9.2	10.0	10.8	11.6
110	242	2.4	2.7	3.4	4.2	4.9	5.6	6.3	7.1	7.8	8.5	9.3	10.0	10.7
120	264	2.3	2.7	3.3	4.0	4.7	5.3	6.0	6.7	7.3	8.0	8.7	9.3	10.0

TABLE 5. ENERGY EXPENDITURE IN METS DURING STEPPING AT DIFFERENT RATES ON STEPS OF DIFFERENT HEIGHTS.

Step Height		Steps per min.			
(cm)	*(in)*	12	18	24	30
0	0	1.2	1.8	2.0	2.4
4	1.6	2.1	2.5	2.9	3.7
8	3.2	2.4	3.0	3.5	4.5
12	4.7	2.8	3.5	4.1	5.3
16	6.3	3.1	4.0	4.7	6.1
20	7.9	3.4	4.5	5.4	7.0
24	9.4	3.8	5.0	6.0	7.8
28	11.0	4.1	5.5	6.7	8.6
32	12.6	4.4	6.0	7.3	9.4
36	14.2	4.8	6.5	8.0	10.3
40	15.8	5.1	7.0	8.7	11.7

METS may be estimated from the work load performed (Tables 4, 5, and 6) or by calculating oxygen intake from measurements of minute ventilation and expired gas composition. Either estimate of METS may be used effectively in exercise prescription.

6. The exercise test should be graded. The initial work load should not exceed 2 to 3 METS for high risk or poorly conditioned participants. The progressive increases in work load should be gradual and usually no

more than 1 MET per step for persons at risk or 2 METS per step for "normals." The graded exercise test may be either continuous or discontinuous in nature. In continuous tests each work level should be performed for at least 1 minute. In discontinuous tests each work load should be performed for approximately 5 minutes with 2 or more minutes of rest between work loads. Data obtained using different exercise test protocols may not be directly comparable.

7. The most objective criterion for the performance of a maximum effort during a graded exercise test is the attainment of maximum oxygen intake. Maximum oxygen intake is attained when with further work rate increments oxygen intake does not increase. Physically conditioned persons can reach a maximum oxygen intake routinely, but sedentary persons and patients reach maximum oxygen intake with difficulty or are unable to reach it. If the graded exercise test is stopped by the physician or exercise technician because of the appearance of a patient's discomfort or other contraindications to exercise, maximum oxygen intake will not likely be attained. Even at the point of exercise limiting fatigue, most poorly conditioned persons will not display a plateau in oxygen intake. In spite of this, an endpoint in graded exercise determined by personal discomfort, severe fatigue, or contraindications observed by the physician or exercise technician is useful as both an evaluative technique and an exercise prescription. This is the maximum level of exercise tolerable to the participant or identified as safe for him by objective criteria. This maximum intensity of graded exercise achieved by a participant and estimated in METS will be called the functional capacity.

TABLE 6. APPROXIMATE RELATIVE ENERGY EXPENDITURE IN METS DURING WALKING OR RUNNING TREADMILL TESTS

Grade		Speed of Walking							
%	km/h	2.7	3.2	4.0	4.8	5.5	5.6	6.4	6.8
	mph	1.7	2.0	2.5	3.0	3.4	3.5	4.0	4.2
0		1.7	2	2.5	3	3.4	3.5	4.6	5
2.5		2.3	2.7	3.3	4	4.5	4.7	6	6.5
5.0		2.9	3.4	4.2	5	5.7	5.9	7.3	7.9
7.5		3.4	4	5	6	6.9	7.1	8.7	9.3
10.0		4	4.7	5.9	7	8	8.3	10	10.8
12.0		4.5	5.3	6.6	7.9	9	9.2	11.1	11.9
12.5		4.6	5.4	6.8	8	9.2	9.5	11.4	12.2
14.0		4.9	5.8	7.3	8.7	10	10.2	12.2	13
15.0		5.2	6.1	7.6	9	10.3	10.7	12.8	13.6
16.0		5.4	6.4	8	9.5	10.8	11.1	13.3	14.2
17.5		5.8	6.8	8.5	10	11.5	11.8	14.1	15
20.0		6.3	7.5	9.3	11	12.7	13	15.5	16.5

Grade	km/h	Speed of Running			
%	mph	9.7 6.0	11.3 7.0	12.9 8.0	14.5 9.0
0		10	11.5	12.8	14.2
2.5		11.4	12.7	14.1	15.4
5.0		12.7	14	15.4	16.7
7.5		13.9	15.3	16.6	18
10.0		15.2	16.5	17.9	19.3
12.5		16.5	17.8	19.2	20.5

A commonly used test is to have the subject walk at 3 mph with 2.5% grade increments utilized each 2 minutes. To convert from mph to km/h, multiply by 1.6093.

8. The ECG should be monitored continuously from at least one chest lead at rest before exercise, during exercise, and in recovery from exercise. A permanent record of the ECG should be obtained at rest, at the end of each level of exercise and in recovery. The blood pressure should be measured at rest, during exercise and during recovery. Monitoring of ECG and blood pressure during the recovery period should be continued until heart rates and blood pressures have stabilized. During the early part of the recovery period the participant should be at supine rest or should exercise at low intensity (zero load 50 to 60 RPM on the bicycle; 2 mph, 0% grade on treadmill, or stepping forward and backward at 24 steps/min). The participant *should not be kept motionless* in the standing position.

9. Effects of Medication on the Exercise Stress Test ECG. Certain medications are known to alter the ECG response to exercise. *False positive tests* may occur in the absence of significant ischemic heart disease when ST–T wave changes result from ingested digitalis preparations or diuretics which have induced hypokalemia. *False negative tests* where ST–T changes are masked may result from treatment with propranolol, quinidine, or reserpine.

Whether or not medications should be temporarily discontinued for graded exercise testing depends on the purpose of the test. If the test is *diagnostic,* it is advisable to remove all confounding medications for sufficient time prior to stress testing to eliminate their possible influence (Appendix C). Alternatively, the exercise might be carried out with the patient continuing his medication and repeated only if expected ischemic ECG changes do

TABLE 7. EMERGENCY EQUIPMENT AND DRUGS

1. Defibrillator (Portable synchronized DC preferable)	1. Morphine or Meperidine
	2. Nitroglycerin tablets and Amyl Nitrite pearls
2. Oxygenator. Intermittent positive pressure capability	3. Catecholamines Aramine Epinephrine 1/10,000 IV Norepinephrine IV Isoproterenol IV
3. Airways, oral and endotracheal	
4. Bag-valve-mask hand respirator (Hope Non-rebreathing bag)	4. Antiarrhythmics Lidocaine IV Procainamide IV Propranolol IV/oral
5. Syringes and needles	5. Atropine sulfate
6. Intravenous sets	6. Digoxin, cedilanid-lanatoside C
7. Intravenous stand	
8. Adhesive tape	7. Sodium Bicarbonate solution
9. Laryngoscope (desirable)	8. Dextrose, 5% in water
	9. Lasix (furosemide) IV
	10. Tensilon (edrophonium)

NOTE: Although these items of equipment and drugs are suggested for emergency use, where possible it is more advisable to be organized into a hospital emergency call system. Under these circumstances only mouth-to-mouth resuscitation and closed chest massage would be performed until the emergency unit arrived.

TABLE 8. EXERCISE EMERGENCIES
(To be managed by the physician).

Basic Causes	Diagnosis	Emergency Procedure
I. CARDIAC ARREST		
A. *Ventricular Fibrillation*	B.P. %, No Heart Sounds, No Pulse, ECG: Ventricular Fibrillation.	—Thump on Chest —Countershock —External Massage
B. *Ventricular Standstill*	B.P. %, No Heart Sounds No Pulse, ECG: Straight Line With P Waves Only.	—Thump on Chest —External Massage —I.V. Adrenalin —External or Internal Pacemaker
II. LOW CARDIAC OUTPUT STATES		
A. *Inadequate Venous Return*	Tachycardia, Low B.P., Pallor, Dizziness	—Supine with Legs Elevated —Isometric or Low Level Isotonic Exercise —Vasopressor Medication
B. *Dysrhythmia* Tachycardia	Must Define by ECG.	Stop Exercise, Supine position,

Bradycardia Irregular	Must Define by ECG. Must Define by ECG.	Treat for inadequate venous return. Ultimately specific treatment depending on ECG diagnosis.
C. *Myocardial Failure*	Inordinate Dyspnea, Pulmonary Rales, Gallop Rhythm.	Stop Exercise, Sitting position, Tourniquets (rotating) and Oxygen breathing.
D. *Drug Induced Low Output* *Propranolol* *Guanethidine*		
III. ISCHEMIC STATUS A. *Myocardial Infarct*	Chest Pain, Unrelenting ECG Evidence.	Stop Exercise, Immediate Hospitalization
B. *Papillary Muscle Dysfunction*	Loud Systolic Murmur—New	—Sitting Position —Nitroglycerin
C. *Cerebral*	Ataxia, Dizziness, Impaired Consciousness	Stop Exercise, Supine Rest
D. *Gastrointestinal*	Nausea, Vomiting, Vasovagal Syncope	Stop Exercise, Supine Rest, Emesis Basin

Cardiovascular collapse: A general term applied to an impairment of cardiovascular function of such severity that the subject cannot stand or walk. This table does not include those symptoms/signs which may occur during exercise testing or training which *do not* result in cardiovascular collapse.

not appear and might have been "masked," or if an unexpected aberration occurs which might have been produced by the medication. For example, if the suspected ischemia did appear despite propranolol, or the ST segment was unequivocally normal with the patient on digoxin, the test need not be repeated. Most ambulatory outpatients can safely be taken off medication for the required washout periods provided adequate medical supervision is available during this interim period and reinstitution of necessary medication follows soon thereafter.

If the test is non-diagnostic and is being done for *functional evaluation* once the diagnosis has been established, it is not necessary to discontinue the medication. Follow-up testing of CHD patients or tests done for exercise prescription are examples. If an individual is to condition while on medication, he should be tested on those medications.

10. Emergency Procedures. Emergency procedures should be carefully organized to ensure maximum safety. An outline of emergency treatment must predetermined and all personnel should have specific duties assigned. Assignments should be written out and available in the laboratory and recreational areas. Emergency equipment and drugs (Table 7) must be available in the immediate area or through a mobile emergency unit and a telephone code system. Laboratory and recreational personnel should be trained in the recognition of an emergency and their appropriate response (Table 8), and in their emergency assignments (see Behavioral Objectives). Procedures should be practiced regularly to drill individuals in their appropriate roles and to maintain and/or improve teamwork.

Guidelines for Exercise Prescription

The prescription of exercise follows certain basic guidelines that are applicable to all individuals regardless of their age, state of health, or their functional capacity. To be meaningful, the exercise prescription must include the type(s) of physical activity, the intensity, the duration, and the frequency. If one exercises, clearly one has an exercise prescription. The prescription, which may be self-prescribed or prescribed by another, may have been developed with great care or with little or no thought or planning.

For someone accustomed to regular exercise minor changes in intensity and duration of the exercise program are a relatively simple matter. Since the participant is aware of what he can do and has some awareness of what he is undertaking, the personal risk is minimal. The risk of even substantial sudden changes in exercise programs is also minimal for healthy, physically active young people. The task of exercise prescription is much more difficult for sedentary, older people, who have risk factors, and particularly those who are symptomatic. Thus, for the individual the degree of risk involved in exercise is likely a function of the interaction of: 1) the severity of the exercise relative to the habitual intensity of exercise performed, 2) age, 3) functional capacity, 4) health, 5) risk factors, and 6) symptomatology. In summary, it is reasonable and not hazardous for many persons to prescribe their own exercise programs, but for others a graded exercise test is highly advisable to ensure a safe and appropriate exercise prescription. The degree of sophistication in the screening before and supervision and monitoring during the graded exercise test will depend on the number and severity of the factors that enhance the risk of the individual during exercise. The range of supervision may vary from mass population testing by unsupervised self-administered step-tests for persons clearly not at risk to graded exercise tests in which heart rate, ECG, blood pressure, oxygen intake, and cardiac output are measured under the supervision of a physician. In graded exercise tests under the direct supervision of trained personnel the minimal criteria for the administration of a safe test are the monitoring of heart rate, blood pressure, and ECG. The maximum safe exercise intensity is determined by the estimation or measurement of the functional capacity in METS (see page 16). Supervised programs or even intermittently supervised programs have the advantage of providing constant feedback on the appropriateness of the prescription for the individual.

A. TYPE OF EXERCISE

Regardless of the type of exercise, each exercise session should be preceded by warm-up exercises of increasing intensity and followed by cooling down exercises of diminishing intensity. The selection of specific activities will be made on the basis of the individual's functional capacity, physical activity interests, the availability of equipment and facilities, and the objectives of the conditioning program. The exercise leader should also utilize a diversity of activities to maintain a balanced program. A balanced program has benefits from both a psychological and physiological viewpoint. The various types of physical activity may be conveniently grouped in terms of their contribution to the objectives of the conditioning program into: 1) Cardiorespiratory Endurance, 2) Flexibility and Relaxation, and 3) Muscular Strength and Endurance.

1. Cardiorespiratory Endurance Activities. The primary concern of the exercise prescription is the development and maintenance of an adequate and stable functional capacity. Therefore, this type of activity will make up the bulk of the exercise program except in unusual circumstances. Functional capacity is enhanced and maintained most effectively by exercises that involve large muscle groups in low tension: high repetition contractions of a rhythmic aerobic nature.

For exercise prescription, cardiorespiratory endurance activities may be classified into three categories: 1) physical activities during which the exercise velocity is easily prescribed and maintained and the individual variability of the cost in METS for a given exercise velocity is small (*e.g.* walking, jogging, running, cycling and distance skating); 2) physical activities during which the exercise velocity is easily maintained but exercise prescription is complicated by wide variations of the cost in METS of performing at a given exercise velocity (*e.g.* swimming and cross-country skiing); and 3) physical activities during which the exercise intensity varies and a given exercise intensity is not maintained (*e.g.* dancing, figure skating, mountain hiking, and a variety of games and sports). Walking, jogging, running, cycling, and distance skating are particularly useful in the early stages of a conditioning program when precise control of effort is necessary to ensure that participants do not get into difficulty by expending too much effort. These activities continue to be useful at all stages of a conditioning program because they enable the participant to expend the most energy per unit time. Furthermore, improvements, plateaus, or regression in performance can be evaluated quickly and efficiently.

Swimming and cross-country skiing are similar to the preceding activities in the degree of control that can be exercised over velocity but the individual variability requires that the energy cost of performing at a given velocity must be determined. Dancing, figure skating, mountain hiking, and a variety of games and sports are effective in providing balance in the exercise program but the prescription, maintenance, and monitoring of intensity are much more difficult (Table 9). They can be extremely useful because of the enjoyment they provide in a physically active setting. Enjoyable activities direct the attention of the participants away from anxieties and worries. However, competitive activities are not recommended for the sedentary or high risk individual. Furthermore, some activities may create their own specific problems. For example, the static effort involved in water skiing or the fatiguing effect of hypoxia and rough terrain during mountain climbing. When games are used as part of the program, they should be supervised and modified carefully to minimize the competitive elements. These activities should not be included until the exercise leader becomes familiar with the exercise tolerance of the individual and the individual's functional capacity is at least 5 METS.

TABLE 9. LEISURE ACTIVITIES: SPORTS, EXERCISE CLASSES, GAMES, DANCING APPROXIMATE RANGE IN ENERGY COST (METS).

	METS		METS
Archery (target or field)	3–4	Horseshoe pitching	2–3
Back Packing	5–11	Hunting (bow or gun)	3–7
Badminton	4–9	Small game (walking, carrying light load)	3–7
Basketball		Hunting (bow or gun)	
Non-game	3–9	Big game (dragging carcass, walking)	3–14
Game Play	7–12	Jogging (running)	
Bed Exercise (arm movement supine or sitting)	1–2	(see Table 6 for speeds)	7–15
Bicycling (pleasure or to work)	3–8	Mountain climbing	5–10
Bowling	2–4	Paddleball (or racquetball)	8–12
Canoeing, rowing and kayaking	3–8	Sailing	2–5
Conditioning exercises (calisthenics)	3–8	Scuba diving	5–10
Dancing (social and square)	3–7	Shuffleboard	2–3
Fencing	6–10	Skating, ice and roller	5–8
Fishing		Skiing, snow	
From bank, boat or ice	2–4	Downhill	5–8
Stream (wading)	5–6	Cross-country	6–12
Football, touch	6–10	Skiing, water	5–7
Golf		Sledding (and tobogganing)	4–8
Using power cart	2–3	Snowshoeing	7–14
Walking (carrying bag or pulling cart)	4–7	Squash	8–12
		Soccer	5–12
Handball	8–12	Softball	3–6
Hiking, cross-country	3–7	Stair-climbing	4–8
Horseback riding	3–8	Swimming	4–8
		Table Tennis	3–5
		Tennis	4–9
		Volleyball	3–6

2. Flexibility and Relaxation Activities. Flexibility exercises can be useful in extending and maintaining the range of movement of a joint or a series of joints. Flexibility exercises should be performed slowly with a gradual progression to greater ranges of motion. Dynamic and static movements may be combined by following a slow ballistic movement with momentarily held static stretch. Although maintenance of flexibility in all joints is important, the lower back is particularly susceptible to chronic soreness and pain. Low back problems may be alleviated by strengthening the abdominal muscles, improvements in posture, and regular stretching exercises for the lower back and the hamstring muscles.

Exercises can also be designed to relieve tension in specific muscle groups. The subject must first be trained to identify the location of muscle groups under tension. Relaxation of the muscle group may be achieved by first contracting the muscle group vigorously while breathing freely and then consciously attempting a complete relaxation. Yoga type exercises are also helpful in the attainment of relaxation. Flexibility and relaxation exercises are effective activities during the warming up and cooling down periods.

3. Muscular Strength and Endurance Activities. Many leisure and occupational tasks require lifting or holding a constant load. Since the strain induced is proportional to the percentage of maximum strength involved, the maintenance or enhancement of muscle strength and muscle endurance will enable the individual to perform such tasks with a minimum of stress. Muscular strength exercises are performed with high tension:low repetition contractions of either a dynamic or static nature.

Static contractions are of limited use since they appear to enhance strength only in the position performed. Furthermore, prolonged static holds or repetitious high tension movements of a total body straining type should be avoided. For people with reduced cardiac adaptability such exercises can be a serious hazard. Dynamic strengthening exercises should be included in a conditioning program. Subjects should be trained to make all strength movements while breathing freely. They may be excluded in favor of cardiorespiratory endurance activities early in the program and even later in the program they should play a relatively minor role. Special attention should be paid to the proper posture and movements during dynamic strength exercises. Unwarranted stress often leads to orthopedic problems.

Strengthening exercises for asymptomatic and symptomatic sedentary individuals should be gradually introduced under supervision. With progress in conditioning most participants will be able to perform such tasks as carrying groceries, mowing the lawn, raking leaves, cutting wood, and shoveling snow safely. However, attention must be directed toward sufficient warming up and cooling off, rhythmic performance of the necessary movements, correct structural and functional position for lifting movements, and regular breathing without breath-holding.

Muscular endurance exercises are low tension, high repetition contractions of a small muscle group that will not require a major increase in total circulation or respiration. For poorly conditioned subjects muscular endurance exercises are useful in increasing both the strength and endurance of small muscle groups without increasing the work of the heart. Muscular strength and endurance exercises have little direct effect on the functional capacity.

The tailoring of an exercise program to the needs of the individual participant is of critical importance. This may require a variety of modifications of any or all activities. The diversity and degree of the modifications depend both on the needs of the individuals in the program and the ingenuity and imagination of the exercise leader. The overriding criterion is that the modified exercise be safe for the participant.

B. INTENSITY OF EXERCISE

The most difficult problem in designing exercise programs is the prescription of the appropriate exercise intensity. This also requires adequate monitoring to ensure that the maximum safe intensity is not exceeded. The percentage of functional capacity a given individual is able to sustain for a given conditioning period is quite variable. Marathon runners are able to maintain 80% of functional capacity for 2 to 4 hours, but, for most poorly conditioned subjects maintenance of 80% would result in exhaustion in less than 30 minutes. Consideration must be given to the fact that the capacity for performing routine or conditioning work is relatively *less* in persons with low functional capacities (6 METS or less) than it is in those with high functional capacities. Reasonable estimates for exercise prescription are that during conditioning sessions peak efforts should not exceed 90% of functional capacity and the average intensity during a conditioning session should approximate 70%. The duration can then be set empirically on the basis that the participant recovers fully and feels rested and not fatigued within an hour following exercise. The exercise program must not only be individually prescribed, but also monitored carefully to ensure that the intensity and duration elicit a conditioning response but do not constitute a risk to the health of the participant. The intensity of the exercise may be prescribed by METS or by heart rate.

1. Exercise Prescription by METS. The peak and average intensity of exercise may be estimated by determining 90% and 70% of the individual's functional capacity. For a person with a maximum functional capacity of 8 METS:

Peak Conditioning Intensity $= .9 \times 8 = 7.2$ METS

Average Conditioning Intensity $= .7 \times 8 = 5.6$ METS

There is an alternative method that sets a sliding scale for estimating the average conditioning intensity. The sliding scale allows for the variability due to known differences in the intensity that can be tolerated by persons with different functional capacities. The baseline intensity is set at 60% of the functional capacity in METS. Thus, for persons with functional capacities ranging from 3 to 20 METS:

Functional Capacity (METS)	Percentage plus Functional Capacity	Average Conditioning Intensity (METS)
3	60 + 3 = 63	1.90
5	60 + 5 = 65	3.25
10	60 + 10 = 70	7.00
15	60 + 15 = 75	11.25
20	60 + 20 = 80	16.00

The average exercise intensity during a given conditioning session does not have to be of continuous work but could be modified frequently by using discontinuous work, *i.e.,* alternating periods of work at higher and lower intensities. If, for example, an exercise intensity of 5.5 METS is prescribed, equal time intervals at 4 and 7 METS will result in the prescribed 5.5 MET average. Thus, any desirable and feasible modification can be prescribed rather precisely. The high intensity period is presumably more likely to be hazardous and, therefore, this format should be approached with great caution.

In most cases, the conditioning effect allows individuals to increase the total work done per exercise session. In continuous work this occurs by an increase in intensity, duration, or some combination of the two. If an individual is doing discontinuous work, the possibilities for increasing total work are more numerous because of the different opportunities for increasing the average intensity. The physician or program director will have to make changes in the exercise prescription as these training effects occur. Periodic reevaluations which may include graded exercise testing will help in reassessment.

For quite a few physical activities such as walking, jogging, running, bicycle ergometer work, and stepping or stair climbing, the exercise intensity in METS is directly related to the speed of movement or to the measurable resistance to overcome. However, the maintenance of the prescribed safe conditioning intensity can be complicated by changes in the environment. Critical environmental factors include: wind; hills; sand; snow; obstacles such as ditches, fences, underbrush; heat or

TABLE 10. NON-SPORTS LEISURE ACTIVITIES APPROXIMATE RANGE IN ENERGY COST (METS).

	METS
Carpentry	2–7
Electric vibrator	2
Gardening	
Hoeing	4–8
Digging, shoveling and pushing	4–8
Wheelbarrow	4–10
Weeding	3–5
Raking	3–6
Home Improvement (painting, plumbing, etc.)	3–8
Heavy Housework (scrubbing floors, making beds, etc.)	3–6
Light Housework (sweeping, polishing, ironing, etc.)	2–4
Mowing lawn	
On cart	2
Power mower	4–5
Hand mower	4–6
Splitting and sawing wood or cutting trees	
Hand	5–10
Power	2–4
Snow shoveling	
Wet snow	8–15
Powder snow	6–9
Walking (see Table 6 for speeds)	
Horizontal or slight grade	3–5
Steep grade	6–8
Upstairs	6–8
Downstairs	4–5

cold; high humidity or high altitude; bulky clothing (*e.g.* vapor barrier clothing), clothing that obstructs movement; and the weight of equipment such as back packs, skis, suitcases, grocery bags, etc.

Prescription and maintenance of safe exercise levels are even more difficult in complex individual sports of swimming, skiing, rowing; dual sports such as tennis, handball or squash; and team sports such as volleyball, softball, soccer, or touch football (Table 10). However, the problem of working at a prescribed training intensity in any activity under any environmental conditions

TABLE 11. OCCUPATIONAL ACTIVITIES. APPROXIMATE RANGE IN ENERGY COST (METS).

Sitting: Light or moderate work (1½–4½ METS)

   a. Sitting at desk writing, calculating, etc.
   b. Driving a car
   c. Using hand tools, light assembly work, radio repair, etc.
   d. Just driving a truck
   e. Working heavy levers, dredge, etc.
   f. Sitting for crane operation
   g. Driving heavy truck or trailer rig (must include getting on and off frequently and doing some arm work)

Standing: Moderate work (2½–5½ METS)

   a. Standing quietly, assembling light or medium machine parts where speed is not a factor; working at own pace or a moderate rate. Can be using light hand tools

TABLE 11. OCCUPATIONAL ACTIVITIES *(Continued)*

b. Just standing, just bartending
c. Using hand tools (gas station operator, other jobs where these are used other than assembly work all day)
d. Scrubbing, waxing, polishing (floors, walls, cars, windows)
e. Assembling or repairing heavy machine parts such as farm machinery, plumbing, airplane motors, etc.
f. Light welding
g. Stocking shelves, packing or unpacking small or medium objects, stocking grocery store shelves
h. Sanding floors with a power sander
i. Assembling light or medium machine parts on assembly line or working with tool or tools on line when objects appear at an appropriate rate of 500 times a day or more (for example, brick laying, plastering, etc.)
j. Working on assembly line when parts require lifting at about every five minutes or so, lifting involves only a few seconds at a time, parts weigh 45 lb. or less
k. Same as above, parts weigh over 45 lb.
l. Cranking up dollies, hitching trailers, operating large levers, jacks, etc.
m. Pulling on wires, twisting cables, jerking on ropes, cables, etc., such as rewiring houses
n. Masonry, painting, paperhanging

Walking: Moderate Work (2½–5½ METS)

a. Walking
b. Carry trays, dishes, etc.

TABLE 11. OCCUPATIONAL ACTIVITIES *(Continued)*

   c. Walking involved in gas station mechanic work (changing tires, wrecker work, etc.)

Standing and/or Walking: Heavy Arm Work (2½–10½ METS)

                                         Mean value in parentheses below

  a. Lifting and carrying objects
      1. 20– 44 lb. (9–20 kg) (4.5)
      2. 45– 64 lb. (20–29 kg) (6.0)
      3. 65– 84 lb. (30–38 kg) (7.5)
      4. 85–100 lb. (39–45 kg) (8.5)
  b. Heavy tools
      1. Pneumatic tools (jackhammers, drills, spades, tampers) (6.0)
      2. Shovel, pick, tunnel bar (8.0)
  c. Moving, pushing heavy objects, 75 lb. or more
      1. These can be desks, file cabinets, heavy stock furniture, such as moving van work. Also include here pushing against heavy spring tension as in boiler room, etc. (8.0)
  d. Other Responses
      1. Laying railroad track (7.0)
      2. Cutting trees—chopping wood (3.0)
         a. Automatically (3.0)
         b. Hand axe or saw (5.5)
  e. Carpentry
      1. Hammering, sawing, planing (6.0)
  f. General heavy industrial labor
      1. Handyman work, some moving, some heavy work as shovel, carpentry, etc.

may be solved by using heart rate as a readily available indicator of energy expenditure.

2. *Exercise Prescription by Heart Rate.* In general, when tachycardia producing psychological stimuli is low, there is a nearly linear relationship between metabolic demands and heart rate or pulse frequency. Existing individual differences will be detected during the graded exercise test. The slope of the line between the individual's resting and exercise heart rates is established in relation to the energy demands. The "maximal" heart rate is the heart rate measured at the level of the safe functional capacity. If one plots the test data, with METS on the abscissa and heart rate on the ordinate, the heart rate pertaining to a given percent level of functional capacity can readily be obtained. This heart rate value, called the target heart rate, may be used for estimating intensity during conditioning. An alternative method is to determine the target heart rate for a conditioning program by multiplying the difference between the maximum and resting heart rates by the same percentage as was used to determine the exercise prescription in METS. This value is then added to the resting heart rate to obtain the target heart rate. For example, if a subject has a resting heart rate of 60 and a maximum heart rate of 180, the available heart rate range is 120 beats/min. With a functional capacity of 10 METS, the prescription calls for a conditioning intensity of 70% of functional capacity, that is 7 METS. The target heart rate then would be 70% of the available H.R. range plus the resting H.R., *i.e.* $(120 \times .7) + 60 = 144$ beats/min.

During some physical activities, the heart rate-MET relationship may be different than during the conditions of the graded exercise test. However, these differences are not great and furthermore the heart rate is possibly the best single indirect measure of the work rate of the heart. Therefore, the target heart rate calculated by the procedures outlined above is applicable, for all practical purposes, to all the physical activities the individual may engage in and to all environmental conditions under which these physical activities may be performed.

In discontinuous work the alternating higher and lower energy demands may be accompanied by heart rates 10% higher or 10% lower than the prescribed target heart rate. However, the work intervals should be of such duration that the heart rate, over time, averages out at the prescribed level.

Heart rate can be determined by ECG monitoring, radiotelemetry or palpation. The latter two methods are more adaptable to non-laboratory situations, with the palpation technique better suited for large groups. Counting the pulse for either 10 or 15 seconds immediately after a bout of exercise gives a good estimation of working heart rate.

In a specific physical conditioning session, the exercise leader may use MET prescription, heart rate prescription or both in setting appropriate exercise levels in various activities. As one adapts to conditioning, heart rate for a given MET load will generally decrease, therefore, participants will be able to progressively increase their MET load to correspond to their target heart rate. Again, periodic reevaluation will aid in measuring progress and checking the exercise prescription.

C. DURATION OF EXERCISE

Throughout this section the duration of exercise will not include the warm-up or cool-down time. The duration of exercise is inversely related to the intensity of the exercise expressed as a percentage of functional capacity. Compared to persons with low functional capacity, persons with high functional capacity are also able to maintain a higher percentage of their functional capacity for a longer period of time. The conditioning response resulting from an exercise program is a function of the interaction of the intensity and the duration of exercise. Significant cardiovascular improvements have been obtained with exercise sessions of 5 to 10 minutes' duration with an intensity of more than 90% of functional capacity. However, high intensity–short duration sessions are not desirable for most participants and better results are obtained with lesser intensities and longer durations.

For normal subjects, exercise sessions of moderate duration (20 to 30 minutes) and moderate intensities (60 to 70% of functional capacity) are advisable during the first weeks of conditioning. Changes in the exercise prescription may be made as the individual's functional capacity increases and as the exercise leader and the individual gain a better understanding of his tolerance for exercise. Modification of the duration–intensity level should be individualized on the basis of the subject's functional capacity, health status, and response to specific exercise activities. If a normal conditioning response is obtained with no complications, the duration should be increased to 20 to 45 minutes after the first few weeks.

As mentioned in the section on intensity, the interaction of intensity and duration should be such that the participant is fully recovered an hour after the exercise session.

An adequate conditioning response can be elicited by maintaining a prescribed work intensity, or a prescribed heart rate, for a period of about 15 minutes per exercise session. With the inclusion of the important "warm-up" and "cool-down" periods the total duration per session would usually run up to 25 to 30 minutes. In many cases daily exercise of such duration will result in the achievement and maintenance of a desirable level of functional capacity.

With a reduction of exercise sessions from four to three or to two per week, the duration of each session should be increased. The duration of a conditioning session should be inversely related to the prescribed exercise intensity as well as to the frequency of weekly exercise sessions. This means that persons with very low functional capacities must tolerate longer conditioning periods. The increase of exercise duration at the lower levels of prescribed exercise appears paradoxical but in practice, such a prescription has proved effective in the improvement of functional capacity. However, almost any exercise prescription has to be individually modified according to specific physical conditions and health problems. As a rule, in the initial stage of a conditioning program the work intensity should be about 1 MET lower than estimated and the total duration of actual exercise should be shortened. This can be most readily achieved by alternating work periods of short duration at the prescribed intensity with sufficiently long recovery periods, not altering the total time the individual is supposed to spend in the supervised program. Under clinical conditions, in the early stage of recuperation from a disease, such type of interval training may call for very short periods of very light exercise and long periods of rest in between. The necessity for individual modifications cannot be overemphasized.

The prescription and supervision of exercise programs for patients are entirely the responsibility of the physician consulting with the exercise leader. No attempt can be made to provide a list of all the possible modifications for certain situations.

Major modifications in intensity and duration of exercise may be required for symptomatic patients and for persons after long periods of bed rest due to illness or surgery. Patients with symptoms of exertional angina may have to exercise for a brief period at only 40 to 50% of functional capacity when initiating an exercise program. Eventually, work intensity and duration can be progressively increased to a level which can be maintained for a longer period of time. As a rule, exercise should not be abruptly stopped when the first warning signs of cardiac limitations become evident but should be continued at a lower intensity to prevent complications created by hydrostatic blood pooling in the lower extremities. Functional capacities are often as low as 2 to 3 METS following a debilitating illness or major surgery. Initially, exercise duration may be restricted to periods of less than 5 minutes due to local muscle fatigue, breathlessness, or both. A reasonable intensity and duration can be established on an empirical basis by ensuring that the subject is fully recovered the following day.

D. FREQUENCY OF EXERCISE SESSIONS

The frequency of exercise will depend in part on the duration and intensity of the exercise session. The optimal frequency of sessions may vary from several daily sessions of only a few minutes during early rehabilitation of a severely limited patient, to three to five 20- to 45-minute periods per week. The program director or exercise leader should determine the frequency of exercise for the specific requirements of participants. For individuals with functional capacities less than 3 METS, sessions of less than 5 minutes several times daily may be more desirable. For persons with capacities between 3 and 5 METS who are exercising minimal durations, daily sessions are advisable. Participants who have capacities of 8 METS and above should have exercise sessions at least 3 times a week. If training is less than daily, sessions should be scheduled on alternate days.

E. TYPES OF EXERCISE PROGRAMS

Medical examination and graded exercise testing permit the classification of people according to their capacity for participation in unsupervised or supervised exercise programs.

1. Unsupervised Exercise Programs. The asymptomatic, presumed normal individual with a functional capacity of 8 METS or more can usually exercise safely in an unsupervised conditioning program. However, one may be aided by exercise prescriptions; knowledge of the energy cost of various activities; methods by which to pace oneself; and by the techniques of prescription by METS and by heart rate.

With the attainment of a satisfactory functional response during a graded exercise test and an adequate functional capacity, participants in a formerly supervised program may change to an unsupervised exercise program. The change to a completely self-administered program may be effected in stages with the participant supervised daily, twice weekly, weekly, monthly, and eventually yearly. Persons who have had cardiovascular or other problems should return for at least annual checkups which include a graded exercise test.

2. *Supervised Exercise Programs.* Supervised exercise programs are advisable for asymptomatic, presumed normals with functional capacities less than 8 METS, and for symptomatic patients regardless of their functional capacities. Prior to participation in a supervised exercise program, the participants should sign an informed consent form (Appendix D). Each exercise session might be supervised in some programs; whereas in other programs supervised sessions might be interspersed with unsupervised sessions. When supervised sessions are intermittent, the unsupervised exercise in the intervening time should be carefully prescribed, participants should be trained to monitor their own exercise intensity by METS and heart rate and an exercise log should be kept. Depending upon the functional capacity and health status of the participants, supervised sessions may be held 3 times a week, once a week, or monthly. The supervised exercise program should be under the combined guidance of a physician and the exercise program director. Direct supervision of each session by a physician is not mandatory in a preventive activity program but the attendance of qualified personnel is a primary requirement for

all programs that include participants with suspected or identified coronary heart disease, or any other disease that increases the risk of participation in vigorous exercise.

Every effort should be made to gradually move participants to programs with less and less supervision as soon as it is deemed safe for them to do so. This is achieved most effectively by a gradual transition with less and less supervision. If the participant proves that he is able to self-administer his own program, he is given more and more freedom to do so; however, checkups are advisable on at least an annual basis.

Behavioral Objectives for Physicians, Program Directors, Exercise Leaders and Exercise Technicians

In order to fully understand the rationale for the writing of the behavioral objectives that follow, it is first necessary to define the term. A behavioral objective is a statement indicating what a person should be able to do following some unit of instruction or study. Much confusion has arisen of late concerning the use of behavioral objectives. Probably one of the most common criticisms voiced against the use of behavioral objectives is that the real objectives of education are mental processes (knowledge, understanding, feelings, etc.) as opposed to actual behavior. Mental processes are activities and events that go on within the human organism and are not directly observable.

It is maintained here that behavior and mental processes are not separate entities. Though we cannot visualize the process by which a person analyzes a short story and only see the results or hear a report of his analysis, we do not see a person solve a problem but we do see the results of the solutions to the problem. Hence, the only way that we can say anything with any certainty about the quality of a person's mental processes is through *inferences* made from observable behavior. The strength then of behavioral objectives is that they permit inferences to be made of these mental processes through behavior.

Two types of objectives will be presented here. The first type will be referred to as a *General Objective* (G.O.). It is within this objective that the unobservable mental process is described. The G.O. will contain the following three parts:

A. Learner term—A description of the person who is to perform the task.
B. Process term—A description of the mental process.
C. Content statement—A description of the content of the learning task.

The second type of objective will be referred to as a *Specific Learning Outcome* (S.L.O.). It is in the S.L.O. that behavior is described in observable terms. It is from the S.L.O. that we then can make inferences about the G.O. The S.L.O. will contain the five following parts:

1. Conditions—The stimuli under which the learner is expected to perform; the environmental conditions which may affect performance.
2. Learner term—A description of the person or persons who will be performing the task.
3. Behavioral term—The observable verb term or action word; exactly what the learner is to do.
4. Content statement—A description of the *content* of the learning task.
5. Criteria—A description of the success criteria by which the learner's response will be judged acceptable or unacceptable.

In the following pages, each professional group will have a designated number of G.O.'s that describe mental processes that are considered here as minimal competencies for each group. The successful completion of the S.L.O.'s that follow each G.O. should indicate the achievement of the mental process described in the related G.O.

PHYSICIAN

The role of a physician in an exercise program of prevention, intervention and cardiac rehabilitation is an important one. The physician serves as a leader and also assumes a support role in the program. In the leadership position the physician is a diagnostician, a teacher and counselor. In his support role the physician recognizes the special talents of program directors, exercise leaders and technicians and delegates responsibilities appropriate to their talents. The physician must understand the clinical and diagnostic terminology relating to exercise and the meaning of exercise test data. He must be able to recognize electrocardiographic signs of dysrhythmias, ischemic and injury patterns and evolving patterns of infarction. Furthermore, the physician must be aware of the hazards associated with exercise including the early signs and symptoms of dysfunction before, during and after exercise. As a teacher, the physician should direct and participate in emergency management programs and provide ongoing education for the exercise program staff. Success of the exercise program depends upon communication. The physician's involvement and cooperation are critical.

The physician in an exercise program must be licensed to practice in the jurisdiction involved and should be covered by appropriate professional liability insurance.

1. *Patient Screening*

   G.O. The physician will know correct procedures for screening a patient before exercise testing.

   S.L.O. Given information concerning pre-exercise testing, the physician will describe in writing the organization and procedures of pre-exercise testing including:

   A. Medical history.
   B. Physical examination.
   C. Contraindications to testing.
   D. Laboratory data to be obtained.
   E. Written informed consent.

2. *Graded Exercise Test Administration*

   G.O. The physician will know the correct procedures for administration of graded exercise tests.

   S.L.O. Given information concerning administration of graded exercise tests, the physician will:

   A. Describe three progressive exercise test procedures, objectives and the values of the information derived.

   B. Describe at least five procedures for ensuring quality control. This includes data acquisition, the supervision of the application of electrodes and the quality of electrocardiographic recordings.

   C. List at least ten signs and symptoms of circulatory, respiratory, cerebral or musculoskeletal dysfunction or inadequacy and identify the usefulness of such signs and symptoms as criteria which determine alteration or termination of the progressive exercise testing session.

D. Orally describe the organization, direction and teaching required in emergency management program(s) including:

1. Cardiopulmonary resuscitation and related functions.
2. Electrical depolarization (defibrillation).
3. Patient evacuation to appropriate intensive care or other facilities.
4. Evaluation and administration of therapy for the responses and side effects of various drugs that are common in cardiac patients and their relationship to exercise and emergency procedures —samples are:

   Vasodilators: nitroglycerin, isosorbide dinitrate, etc.

   Antihypertensives: guanethidine, alpha methyldopa, hydralazine, reserpine

   Antidysrhythmics: quinidine, procaineamide, propanolol, lidocaine

   Digitalis preparations: digoxin, digitoxin, ouabain

   Hypoglycemics: insulin, phenformin, sulfonylurea, chlorpromazine

   Diuretics: thiazides, furosemide

   Sympathomimetics: Adrenalin, isoproterenol, Noradrenalin, metaraminol bitartrate

Anticoagulants: Coumadin, heparin
Analgesics: codeine, morphine
Parasympatholytic agents: atropine
Steroids: methylprednisolone, predni-
sone, cortisone
Solutions: dextrose, sodium lactate,
Ringer's, sodium bicarbonate

3. *Post Exercise Procedures*
  G.O. The physician will understand post exercise procedures.
  S.L.O. Given five hypothetical situations that may arise
during post exercise examining procedures, the
physician will:
  A. Outline the criteria which determine when
to discontinue direct monitoring of the patient, when to send to showers, etc., and discharge from laboratory.
  B. Interpret observations and results of exercise
testing and summarize findings in the con-
text of a patient's status and desired program.
  C. Describe the importance of communicating
results to referring physician(s) or institu-
tion and/or patient if requested by a referring source.
  D. Describe exercise prescriptions including in-
structions on safeguards and precautions
and how to vary workload appropriate to
temperature, humidity, recent illness and
disabilities.
  E. Describe the procedures of providing ap-

propriate support and advice to patients in a program as requested, with close communication with the patient's physician(s) and appropriate triage to them of new circumstance.

F. Outline the criteria which determine schedules for re-evaluation and/or interim examination relative to patient status and change in status.

4. *Staff Education*

G.O. The physician will understand the importance of staff education.

S.L.O. Given the responsibility as a medical supervisor of a cardiac rehabilitation program and a support staff consisting of exercise leaders and technicians, the physician will:

A. Orally describe the significance and implications of risk factors, stress testing, laboratory data and scientific study results with regard to physical training, health enhancement and rehabilitation.

B. Orally describe safety program(s) to include necessary instruction of all personnel, maintenance of equipment and periodic evaluation to reduce hazards and maintain competence in preventive and emergency services.

PROGRAM DIRECTOR

Exercise appears to have a legitimate and accepted role in both preventive and rehabilitative medical programs. As a result, there is an increasing demand for information about exercise testing and physical conditioning programs by the medical and health-related professions. In order to meet this demand, more and more highly qualified, specially trained exercise specialists are needed.

Because the exercise specialist who becomes a program director must meet the requirements of the exercise technician and exercise leader, most probably he will have had much of the practical background necessary for the testing and physical conditioning portions of the program. However, in order to understand the medical and physiological implications of the tests and the resulting exercise programs and in order to understand how and why certain activities are recommended or contraindicated, more theoretical experience is needed. Hopefully, the majority of this knowledge will have been obtained during his studies for an advanced degree in physical education, physiology or medicine.

Since the program director is responsible for: 1) the inclusion of adequate exercise testing procedures; 2) accurate, individualized prescription of activities; and 3) careful supervision and leadership of a safe, effective and enjoyable exercise program, he needs the theoretical and practical backgrounds associated with certain aspects of medicine, physiology, physical education and behavioral psychology. Thus, he is a unique specialist in that he must draw from a wide range of abilities, knowledges and experiences as they relate to exercise.

The exact role of the program director depends on such factors as his own personal interests, the size of the program and the type of people who will be tested and exercised. If the program is small, then he will probably be involved in the collection and analysis of data obtained during exercise testing and/or the supervision and leadership of the actual exercise programs. If the program is relatively large, then his duties may be primarily administrative and related to the actual prescription of the activity program in close cooperation with the physician. Working with the physician, his duties will also include the training, continuing education and supervision of personnel who work with him, *i.e.,* the exercise technicians and exercise leaders should understand the basic aspects of the physiology of exercise and training, sociopsychological aspects of behavior modification, emergency procedures, particular problems of special groups of patients, etc.

A program director must also work with and communicate with the public, those persons who are tested and exercised in his program, as well as with physicians and health professionals, *i.e.,* with people who have varying degrees of knowledge and sophistication regarding the medical, physiological, psychological and educational aspects of exercise programs. Because of this, he should understand and be able to explain and discuss both the theoretical and practical aspects of exercise and conditioning with each of these various groups of people.

In special programs for middle-aged or older persons, for persons who have a high risk of developing a disease such as coronary heart disease or for those who already have specific medical problems, the program director must understand the medical and physiological implications of the medical history of these patients and provide for any special needs related to the testing, prescription and supervision of exercises. In doing this, he is expected to maintain a close working relationship with the appropriate medical specialist. In such cases where the knowledge and experience necessary to work with these special groups are inadequate and did not form an integral part of his educational background, he is expected to study and learn more about any special aspects of a particular medical or physiological program by means of special courses or symposia, by reading scientific articles and books and by discussions with knowledgeable persons. In other words, he should be a "lifetime student" who continually strives to improve his level of competency within his specialty.

Professional study and cooperation of the program director with physicians, physiologists, physical educators and other health personnel are basic to the optimal realization of health benefits from physical activity programs. This type of team work is especially needed if the benefits from these programs are to be made available to large segments of the public. Obviously, the exercise specialist can and should be a major factor in the success of such a program.

1. *Functional Anatomy*
    G.O. The program director will understand the areas of human functional anatomy and their interrelationships.
    S.L.O. Given a cadaver in a laboratory setting, the program director will:
    A. Identify all the major components of the human skeleton.
    B. Describe, either orally or in writing, the properties and functions of bone.

C. Identify the location of all the major muscle groups.

D. Describe all the properties and functions of muscle and connective tissue.

E. Identify all five diarthrodial joints of the skeleton.

F. Describe all the properties and functions of the above joints.

G. Identify six components of the vascular system.

H. Describe four functions of the vascular system.

I. List five mechanical laws and explain their application to human movement.

J. Identify two basic patterns of human movement.

G.O. The program director will understand the interrelationship of and the application of the areas of functional anatomy in a prescribed exercise program.

S.L.O. Given a wide variety of orthopedic problems in a laboratory setting, the program director will:

A. Describe five common joint abnormalities.

B. Describe traumatic musculoskeletal injuries.

C. Identify a means by which hypertrophy and atrophy of muscle can occur.

D. List the approximate ranges of motion for the following joints:

1. ankle   4. spine
2. knee   5. elbow
3. hip   6. shoulder

E. Identify at least five acquired body mechanics problems.

F. Describe a physical method of alleviation of each of the common body mechanical problems listed above.

G. Describe an exercise prescription for treatment of five traumatic injuries to the musculoskeletal system.

H. List ten examples in which exercise is contraindicated in the presence of traumatic injuries to the musculoskeletal system.

I. Describe five physiological principles involved in exercise prescription for common musculoskeletal problems.

J. Explain a change in exercise prescription due to the following acute common musculoskeletal problems:

1. bursitis
2. tendonitis
3. metatarsalgia
4. arthritis
5. stone bruise

2. *Exercise Physiology*

G.O. The program director will understand the structure of muscle.

S.L.O. Given a series of anatomical drawings, the program director will:

A. Describe the structure of muscle in terms of the following:

1. myofilaments
2. myofibrils
3. fibers
4. motor units

B. Identify three types of fibers on the basis of oxidative capacity, glycolytic capacity and speed of contraction.

G.O. The program director will understand the relationship between muscle structure and function.

S.L.O. Given a series of anatomical drawings, the program director will:
  A. Explain contraction of muscle in terms of the sliding filament theory.
  B. Explain an interrelationship among motoneuron size, discharge threshold, frequency and recruitment.
  C. Describe the relationship of motoneuron diameter and motor unit size.

G.O. The program director will understand the mechanics of muscle contraction.

S.L.O. Given a series of laboratory demonstrations, the program director will:
  A. Define twitch, summation and tetanus in terms of muscle contraction.
  B. Draw and explain the relationship between force and velocity of shortening.
  C. Describe one way by which the tension exerted by a muscle might increase or decrease.
  D. Explain the chief difference between an isometric and an isotonic contraction.
  E. Define the biochemistry of muscle fatigue under specified conditions of task, intensity and duration of exercise.
  F. Explain the difference in the fatigability of the three types of muscle fibers in terms of energy pools, energy use and energy resynthesis.

G.O. The program director will understand the concept of a graded exercise test (see behavioral objectives for Exercise Technician, pp. 90–97).

S.L.O. Given a series of protocols, the program director will:

    A. List ten criteria for a safe and valid exercise test for presumed normals and for patients.

    B. List at least five advantages and five disadvantages for each of the following: stepping devices, bicycle ergometry and treadmill testing.

    C. List at least three advantages and three disadvantages of a continuous test.

    D. List at least three advantages and three disadvantages of a discontinuous test.

G.O. The program director will understand the metabolic, respiratory and circulatory response to graded submaximum exercise.

S.L.O. Given a series of submaximal exercise testing results, the program director will:

    A. List normal resting values for heart rate (HR), stroke volume (SV), cardiac output ($\dot{Q}$), (a–v) O_2 difference, O_2 uptake ($\dot{V}O_2$), systolic, diastolic blood pressure (SBP, DBP), minute ventilation ($\dot{V}E$), tidal volume (VT), breathing frequency (f).

    B. Graph the percentage increase in HR, SV, $\dot{Q}$, (a–v) O_2 difference, $\dot{V}O_2$ SBP, DBP, $\dot{V}E$, VT and f relative to the increase in workload expressed as a percentage of maximum physical work capacity.

    C. Describe the mechanism by which each parameter listed in B above increases with increasing work intensity (some mechanisms may not be known).

D. Describe the effect of warming up on the physiological response to exercise and on performance.

E. List at least four differences in the circulatory response of patients with diagnosed CHD compared to that of normals.

F. Graph the return of respiration, circulation and metabolism to resting values during recovery.

G. Describe the physiological effects of cooling down gradually after exercise, specifically, those related to the respiratory and circulatory system.

H. Define MET and calculate the energy cost in METS for given work rates on steps, bicycle ergometer and treadmill.

I. List the approximate energy required to do 1 kg m/min of work, to move 1 kg of body weight horizontally 1 m/min by running, to move 1 kg of body weight horizontally 1 m/min by walking (walking estimate is less accurate because of curvilinear relation between energy cost and velocity).

J. List at least five differences in the circulatory response to static work compared to dynamic work and describe the importance of these differences in exercise prescription.

K. Describe the contribution of aerobic and anaerobic metabolism to the total energy cost of work at 60, 80 and 100% of maximum physical work capacity.

G.O. The program director understands respiratory, circulatory and metabolic response to maximum exercise.

S.L.O. Given a series of maximum exercise testing results, the program director will:

A. Identify maximum oxygen intake (functional capacity).

B. List approximate range of values of functional capacity in METS of endurance athletes, normal untrained adults and cardiac patients,

C. Describe the interaction of HR and SV, and $\dot{Q}$ and $(a-v)$ O_2 difference as $\dot{V}O_2$ reaches a plateau.

D. List maximum values for HR, SV, $\dot{Q}$, $(a-v)$ O_2 difference, $\dot{V}O_2$, $\dot{V}E$, VT, f, SBP for untrained and trained adults.

E. Describe the interaction of preload, after load, diastolic filling time and contractility in the increase, plateau and decrease in SV.

G.O. The program director understands the specificity of conditioning and the physiological differences between endurance conditioning and strength conditioning.

S.L.O. Given two sets of objectives in endurance conditioning and strength conditioning, the program director will:

A. Describe specificity of conditioning in terms of tension, number of repetitions, duration, muscle groups involved and type of task.

B. List at least five salient features of an endurance conditioning program and of a strength program.

  C. Explain at least five reasons why endurance and strength conditioning are important in rehabilitation.
  D. List at least three advantages and three disadvantages of an isotonic compared to an isometric conditioning task.
  E. Describe five hazards of a high intensity conditioning program for sedentary adults and/or symptomatic patients.
  F. Outline at least three criteria necessary for a conditioning program to increase functional capacity.

G.O. The program director will understand the concept of the reversibility of conditioning.

S.L.O. Given examples of the physiological profiles of sedentary men, the program director will:
  A. Define atrophy and explain the cause of atrophy.
  B. List a total of five changes that occur in muscle or in the respiratory, circulatory and metabolic response to exercise following a decrease in physical activity, bed rest or casting of a limb of one month's duration.

G.O. The program director will understand the characteristics which differentiate the conditioned from the unconditioned.

S.L.O. Given the progressive exercise testing results, age, height and weight, the program director will:
  A. List at least three variables which most clearly differentiate between persons with high functional capacity (conditioned) and persons with low functional capacity (un-

conditioned) at rest and in maximum exercise.

B. List a value for each of the three listed above that most clearly differentiate between the conditioned and unconditioned, at rest and maximum exercise.

C. List the percentage increase in functional capacity an unconditioned adult might expect following a conditioning program.

D. Explain the mechanism by which the functional capacity increased during a conditioning program.

G.O. The program director understands the adaptations that occur in skeletal muscle and cardiac muscle during a conditioning program.

S.L.O. Given the performance characteristics of a sedentary man, the program director will:

A. List one adaptation that occurs in skeletal muscle and in heart muscle and explain the adaptation.

B. Explain the effect of the adaptation listed above on performance and on muscle fatigue.

C. Explain two effects of the changes on $\dot{Q}$ and $\dot{V}O_2$ during a conditioning program.

D. Define hypertrophy and explain the stimulus for hypertrophy.

E. Explain the interaction of hypertrophy, capillary density, mitochondrial density and the contractile characteristics of a fiber (fast or slow twitch) on the capacity of a fiber to perform specific tasks (*i.e.,* endurance or strength).

G.O. The program director understands total body metabolism, caloric intake and calorie storage in terms of the concepts of molecular interconvertibility, dynamic steady-states and the first law of thermodynamics.

S.L.O. Given data, to include anthropometry, which indicate a subject's food ingestion and energy expenditure for a 48-hour period of time, the program director will:

A. Define the first law of thermodynamics and apply $E = $ heat $+$ work to the concept of metabolic rate.

B. Describe biological work in terms of external work and internal work.

C. Define basal metabolic (BMR) and resting metabolic rate (RMR) and list normal values for BMR and RMR.

D. Describe three determinants of basal metabolic rate.

E. Describe the control of food intake by hypothalamic integrating centers.

F. Define specific dynamic effect in terms of metabolic cost of five physical activities.

G. Define obesity and describe the primary cause.

H. Describe the interaction between diet and exercise in the maintenance of body weight.

I. Estimate percentage of body weight that is fat by skinfold thickness methods.

J. Describe the differences in the accuracy of

estimates of body fatness by underwater weighing and by skinfold thickness.

G.O. The program director will understand temperature regulation of the body and the effect of environmental factors on regulation.

S.L.O. Given a series of ambient temperatures and humidities, the program director will:

A. List normal values for oral, rectal and skin temperatures in a neutral environment at rest and the range of rectal temperatures compatible with life.

B. Describe the control of body temperature in terms of: hypothalamic thermoreceptors, peripheral thermoreceptors, hypothalamic integrating center, efferent pathways, effector mechanisms as they relate to heat production, heat loss and heat storage.

C. Write the heat balance equation.

D. Describe at least five behavioral aspects of temperature regulation.

E. Use the principles of heat production, heat loss and heat storage to describe temperature regulation at two different work rates performed at two different ambient temperatures.

F. Describe adaptation to heat and to cold.

G. List four factors that contribute to hyperthermia.

H. List critical core temperature (unconsciousness); lethal temperature.

I. List one procedure each for treating a patient suffering from hyperthermia and hypothermia.

J. Define wind-chill index.

K. Define Q-10 effect.

L. Describe the mechanism of fever.

G.O. The program director will understand adaptation to low barometric pressure, the effects of low barometric pressure on the respiratory, circulatory and metabolic response to graded exercise and on maximum oxygen uptake.

S.L.O. Given a series of examples of low barometric pressures, the program director will:

A. List three immediate adaptations to hypoxia (first day).

B. List three subsequent adaptations to hypoxia (3 to 4 days of exposure).

C. List four long term adaptations to hypoxia (year or more).

D. Graph respiratory, circulatory and metabolic response to graded exercise for the normal sea level response.

E. Explain five differences between the hypoxic and sea level response.

F. Graph the percentage decrease in maximum oxygen intake with decreasing barometric pressure.

G. Explain the mechanism by which maximum oxygen intake decreases with decreasing barometric pressure.

H. Describe the five modifications that must be made in endurance training programs at given altitudes.

3. *Pathophysiology*

G.O. The program director will understand the pathophysiology of various cardiovascular, respiratory and metabolic diseases.

S.L.O. Given information concerning coronary anatomy and cardiac physiology the program director will:

A. Draw and identify the major vessels of the coronary circulation.

B. List three factors associated with the development of coronary arteriosclerosis.

C. List two determinants of myocardial oxygen supply.

D. List the three major determinants of myocardial oxygen consumption.

E. Describe two reasons why exercise increases myocardial oxygen consumption.

F. Describe why significant obstruction of the coronary artery(ies) would limit exercise capacity.

G. Describe three indications of myocardial ischemia which may be a cause for terminating a graded exercise test.

H. Describe two physiological changes which would lower myocardial oxygen consumption for a given submaximal work intensity following a physical training program.

I. List one other form of treatment which would lower myocardial oxygen consumption in exercise.

J. Describe a surgical treatment which would increase blood flow to the myocardium.

K. List two indices for estimating myocardial oxygen consumption.

S.L.O. To be able to state verbally a description of the following:

A. Diabetes, the role of insulin, the normal values for fasting plasma glucose and the effect of exercise on insulin requirements.

B. Hyper- and hypothyroidism and their relationship to basal metabolic rate.

C. Gout, its relationship to uric acid, and the normal values for uric acid.

D. Arthritis and the use of anti-inflammatory drugs such as cortisol.

E. Hypertriglyceridemia, hypercholesterolemia, lipoprotein electrophoresis patterns and normal values for each.

G.O. The program director will understand the basic physiological effects of specific drugs used in the treatment of various cardiovascular, respiratory and metabolic diseases.

S.L.O. A. To be able to relate the following specific classes of drugs to the purpose for which each is prescribed:

a. vasodilators such as nitroglycerin.

b. antidysrhythmics such as quinidine or propranolol.

c. antihypertensives such as diuretics and others.

d. hypoglycemics such as insulin.

e. "mood" type drugs such as Elavil.

f. anticoagulants such as Coumadin.

g. sympathomimetics such as isoproterenol and phenylephrine.

h. digitalis preparations such as digitoxin.

B. To be able to describe the effect of exercise on the above classes of drugs and vice versa.

4. *Gerontology*

G.O. The program director will understand the effect of the aging process on the structure and function of man.

S.L.O. Given longitudinal data relating to population studies, including information on the musculoskeletal, cardiorespiratory and central nervous system responses of aging man, the program director will:

A. Describe five common orthopedic problems of older subjects and list three activities which may be selected to avoid aggravation of the disabilities.

B. Describe the change in maximum heart rate with advancing age.

C. Identify the age relationship to the incidence of five ECG abnormalities during exercise in essentially healthy subjects.

D. Describe five limitations and five precautions of exercise prescriptions for those with vision impairments.

E. Describe five limitations and five precautions of exercise prescriptions for those with hearing impairments.

F. Discuss the normal changes from about age 30 to 70 with regard to: strength; functional capacity; mechanical efficiency of walking or riding a bicycle; reaction time (latency) and movement time; resting systolic and diastolic blood pressure; exercise systolic and diastolic blood pressure; rate of recovery from exercise in heart rate and metabolism; maximum ventilation during exercise; resting pulmonary measurements; vital capacity, $FEV_{1.0}$, residual volume, and expiratory and inspiratory reserve volume; flexibility; body composition; coordination; cardiac output (rest and exercise); ventilatory efficiency during exercise; tolerance to heat or cold stress.

G. Discuss the effects of a conditioning program to be expected in older compared to younger adults in the characteristics listed in (F) above.

H. Explain five differences in trainability of old compared to young subjects.

I. Describe at least four psychological changes which characterize most men and women after age 40 and explain how these affect motivation to exercise and the selection of activities.

5. *Human Behavior*

G.O. The program director will understand basic principles of human behavior to include communication, motivation and factors which influence behavior over time.

S.L.O. Given a number of case studies of participants in an exercise rehabilitation program, the program director will:

A. Explain the influence of three positive forces that support behavior over time.

B. Describe four negative forces that serve as barriers to behavior change.

C. Explain how the positive forces that support behavior and the negative forces that serve as barriers to behavior change listed above apply to:
   1. Exercise testing
   2. Exercise prescription
   3. Program adherence

D. List and describe five factors that influence the effectiveness of communication.

E. Define the term "selective perception" and give two examples.

F. List five factors that motivate behavior.

G. Describe five methods of positive reinforcement which influence patterns of behavior.

H. Describe two methods by which individuals may be helped to fit exercise into their daily pattern and life style.

I. List three benefits of exercise in relation to work performance and attitudes toward work.

J. List three positive effects of exercise that can alter a person's perceived health status, specifically, sense of well being and tension.

K. Describe five social-psychological effects of exercise in influencing a person's self-concept and self-esteem as well as his perceived control over his health status.

6. *Exercise Laboratory Techniques*
   G.O. The program director will demonstrate skills and competencies in exercise laboratory techniques.
   S.L.O. See S.L.O.'s for exercise technician.
   G.O. The program director will demonstrate skills and competencies in emergency procedures.
   S.L.O. Given a series of examples which require emergency procedures, the program director will:
   A. Describe three principles and three procedures of emergency care.
      1. Cardiopulmonary resuscitation (heart-lung resuscitation, external cardiac compression, mouth-to-mouth and/or mouth-to-nose ventilation).
      2. Alternative methods of artificial ventilation.
      3. Manual methods of ventilation.
      4. Complications.
   B. Operate equipment in conjunction with cardiorespiratory resuscitation:
      1. Manually operated self-inflating bag, valve, mask units.
      2. Pressure cycled automatic ventilators and/or resuscitators.
      3. External cardiac compression machines (physician only).
      4. Defibrillator (physician only).
   C. Describe the technique of tracheal intuba-

tion and two occasions under which such procedures should be undertaken (physicians and nurses only).

D. List at least five medications (drugs) which should be available during exercise sessions for adult participants and the desired effect of each drug upon a patient during an emergency cardiac condition.

E. Discuss the individual responsibility and legal implications relative to emergency care.

7. *Therapeutic Exercise and Exercise Prescription*

G.O. The program director will demonstrate skills and competencies required of the exercise leader.

S.L.O. See S.L.O.'s for exercise leader.

8. *Program Administration*

G.O. The program director will understand the role of administration as a means of facilitation of the program.

S.L.O. Given the responsibility of establishing an exercise intervention and rehabilitation program, the program director will:

A. Define the term "command responsibility."

B. Diagram an organizational chart and show the line-staff relationships between a program director, advisory board, exercise leader, exercise technician, medical advisor, participant's personal physician and participants.

C. List five functional or operating policies for each of the following:

    1. Accident or injury reporting for minor injuries not requiring immediate medical treatment.

    2. Medical supervision of a high risk exercise program.

    3. Confidentiality of participant records.

    4. Program director's relationship to practicing medical doctors recommending patients to the exercise program.

    5. Emergency procedures.

    6. Continuing education of the staff.

    7. Program evaluation.

    8. Education of the spouse of the patient.

    9. Hiring and firing.

D. Explain the role of an advisory committee in terms of patient accession, fees, staff qualifications and liability.

E. List five procedures from an initial contact to the eventual participation of a recent post MI subject.

F. List four types of records and forms a program director would need, develop and use.

G.O. The program director will understand his legal responsibilities.

S.L.O. Given a series of examples of court cases involving physical exercise programs, the program director will:

A. Define the following terms: tort, negligence, liability, informed consent and contract.

B. Describe four defenses against liability for negligence: examination of risk, acts of

God, contributory negligence and lack of appropriate cause.

G.O. The program director will understand specific activities included in an exercise program, methods of evaluating program effectiveness and factors influencing the selection of activities.

S.L.O. Given a wide variety of physical facilities and equipment, the program director will:

A. List five specific activities to be included in programs where the prescribed work rate level is:
   1. 3 to 7 METS
   2. 8 to 10 METS
   3. 11 to 15 METS

B. List four objective methods of evaluating program effectiveness.

C. List five factors which influence the selection of activities offered.

G.O. The program director will understand the design and safety requirements of physical facilities necessary for exercise programs.

S.L.O. Given 1000 square feet of enclosed floor space, the program director will:

A. Design a testing and laboratory facility to include ergometry (stress testing), participant examination, pulmonary function, hematologic equipment, anthropometry, staff office, dressing and shower room. (Space available 25' × 50' × 10'.)

B. Outline five safety procedures in the use and supervision of:
   1. Swimming pool.

      2. The use of climbing ropes and gymnastic apparatus to include trampolines.

      3. The use of weight lifting equipment.

G.O. The program director will understand the concepts of developing a budget (a budget is a written estimate of anticipated income and expenditures).

S.L.O. Given the example of an exercise program's audit, the program director will:

    A. List ten types of consumable or nontagable supplies used in an exercise program.

    B. Describe the first principles of accounting, "for every debit there is a credit."

    C. List five steps in developing a budget.

G.O. The program director will understand principles of public and human relations.

S.L.O. Given various public relations models, the program director will:

    A. Define public relations, empathy and rapport.

    B. List ten methods of informing the public on physical activity programs of prevention, rehabilitation and intervention.

9. *Internship*

In order to qualify as a program director, an internship of at least one year's duration is necessary. The internship should be under the supervision of an established program director and a competent physician and provide opportunities for competencies in the following areas: administration, program leadership, laboratory procedures and exercise prescription. It is assumed that the preceptor of the internship will work closely with the prospective program director. In addition to the opportunity to demonstrate proficiency, oral and written examinations are an integral part of the learning experience.

EXERCISE LEADER

An exercise leader in activity programs of prevention, intervention and cardiac rehabilitation needs, in addition to knowledge, an ability to work with and enjoy people. In all exercise sessions the leader's goal should be to include some activities of an enjoyable nature. Hopefully, along with the physical work accomplished, enjoyment of physical activity will result in the participant's increased proficiency in a wide variety of physical skills and positive attitudes toward work and play. The cognitive aspects of leading men in physical activity can be learned, but to be successful the exercise leader must also possess a high degree of creativity. To vary the program offerings and to meet individual needs requires the ability to innovate. Intervention and rehabilitation exercise programs require participants not only to make but to adhere to long-range commitments. This challenge can be met if the exercise leader has the ability to apply scientific principles of conditioning. He must also motivate people. Sustained participation over a long period of time requires that exercise programs be well supervised, safe and enjoyable.

The following professional undergraduate curricula lend themselves to further education and preparation for the position of exercise leader: physical education, physical therapy, occupational therapy. The role and responsibility of the exercise leader are as follows: to meet the requirements of the exercise technician, interpret metabolic data from exercise tests, execute the exercise prescription (under guidelines established with physician and program director), educate the patient concerning exercise, evaluate the patient's response to exercise and to interact and communicate with the physician, program director, subjects and patients.

1. *Functional Anatomy*

    G.O. The exercise leader will understand functional anatomy.

  S.L.O. Given anatomical models, the exercise leader will:

        A. Identify the major skeletal muscles and muscle groups on examination.

Abdominal Muscles

External oblique
Internal oblique
Transversus abdominis
Rectus abdominis

Muscles Acting Upon The Shoulder Joint

Pectoralis major
Pectoralis minor
Deltoid
Supraspinatus
Infraspinatus
Teres minor
Teres major
Subscapularis
Latissimus dorsi
Coracobrachialis

Muscles Acting Upon The Elbow Joint

Biceps brachii
Brachialis
Brachioradialis
Pronator teres
Triceps brachii

Muscles Acting Upon The Wrist, Hand and Fingers

Flexor carpi radialis
Extensor carpi ulnaris
Extensor carpi radialis longus
Extensor carpi radialis brevis
Flexor digitorum superficialis
Flexor digitorum profundus
Extensor digitorum
Extensor digiti minimi
Extensor indicis

Gluteal Muscles

Gluteus maximus
Gluteus medius
Gluteus minimus

Posterior Thigh Muscles

Biceps femoris
Semitendinosus
Semimembranosus

Anterior Thigh Muscles

Iliopsoas
Quadriceps femoris
Sartorius
Tensor Fasciae Latae

Medial Thigh Muscles

Pectineus
Adductor longus

Adductor brevis
Adductor magnus
Gracilis

Posterior Muscles of The Leg

Gastrocnemius
Soleus
Plantaris
Popliteus
Flexor digitorum longus
Flexor hallucis longus
Tibialis posterior

Anterior Muscles of the Leg

Tibialis anterior
Extensor digitorum longus
    and peroneus tertius
Extensor hallucis longus

B. Name and locate palpable skeletal landmarks of the extremities and trunk.
   1. Superior Extremity: medial and lateral epicondyle of the humerus, ulna, olecranon process and styloid process.
   2. Inferior Extremity: greater trochanter, tibial tuberosity, medial malleolus, lateral malleolus, tibiocalcaneal ligament, calcaneofibular ligament.
   3. Trunk: spinous processes, suprasternal notch, sternoclavicular joint, and acromioclavicular joint.

4. Describe five differences in mechanics of human locomotion in walking, jogging or running and carrying or moving objects.

2. *Exercise Physiology*

G.O. The exercise leader will understand exercise physiology.

S.L.O. Given laboratory diagrams and the results of progressive exercise tests, the exercise leader will:

A. Draw the heart-circulatory system and describe its primary function to the increased energy demands required during work.

B. Draw the lung-respiratory system and describe its primary function to the increased energy demands required during work.

C. Describe the primary difference between aerobic and anaerobic metabolism.

D. List the approximate proportion of aerobic and anaerobic metabolism involved in: playing golf; jogging-running at 4 mph, 8 mph, 10 mph; playing tennis; swimming 100 to 1,000 yards; running the 100 yard dash; skiing downhill.

E. Explain two test protocols by which maximum O_2 intake determinations may be obtained by stepping devices, bicycle ergometry or motor driven treadmill.

F. Describe two maximum O_2 intake assessments and estimates obtained by field tests.

G. Plot a curve and provide supportive evidence of the relationship of maximum O_2 intake to age for both males and females.

H. Describe five effects of ambient temperature and humidity on human health and work capacity, three implications for human safety and an organ system's response to these conditions.

I. Describe the normal response of ventilation, heart rate and blood pressures to graded exercise.

J. List the energy cost in METS of the following physical activities: walking at: 2 mph 5% grade, 3 mph 17½% grade; running at: 4 mph, 8 mph, 10 mph; playing games such as tennis, golf, handball.

K. Describe three differences between muscular atrophy and muscular hypertrophy.

L. Define the following terms: hyperphagia, dyspnea, hyperemia, ischemia, anemia, respiratory alkalosis, angina pectoris, Valsalva maneuver, cardiac output, hypoxia, orthostatic reaction, respiratory acidosis, METS, stroke volume, arterial pressures, calorimetry, hyperventilation, hyperpnea and hypoventilation.

3. *Behavioral Psychology and Group Dynamics*

G.O. The exercise leader will understand behavioral psychology and group dynamics.

S.L.O. Given a series of hypothetic situations of participants in an exercise rehabilitation program, the exercise leader will:

    A. Explain five physiological responses of man to emotional stress.

    B. Describe four teaching techniques used in conducting rehabilitation programs.

    C. Describe three types of instructional techniques used in an exercise rehabilitation program.

    D. Define the following terms and relate each to the management of an exercise program: aggression, projection, denial, play, identification, hedonism, goal orientation-setting, operant conditioning, rapport, recreation, anxiety, empathy, fear, rationalization, relaxation, opinions-attitudes, motivation, euphoria, depression, rejection and catharsis.

4. *Emergency Procedures* (see Guidelines)

    G.O. The exercise leader will demonstrate skills and abilities in emergency procedures.

S.L.O. See S.L.O.'s for exercise technician.

5. *Therapeutic Exercise and Exercise Prescription*

    G.O. The exercise leader will understand therapeutic exercise and exercise prescription.

S.L.O. Given sufficient medical information, the exercise leader will:

    A. Describe the anatomy and physiology of common orthopedic problems associated with physical activity: myositis ossificans, shin splints, tennis elbow, hamstring strain, metatarsalgia, stress fracture, lordosis, osteochondrosis, bone contusion of the os calcis and infrapatellar bursitis.

B. Prepare sample therapeutic exercise prescription for the aforementioned problems and incorporate the principles of frequency, intensity and duration of exercise in a prescription.

C. List and describe eight physical signs of strain which require a cessation or reduction in the intensity of a participant's exercise session.

D. Describe three exercise programs for participants identified as being deficient in muscle strength of:
1. Abdominal muscles.
2. Erector spinae muscles.
3. Quadriceps muscles.

E. Name three procedures and the equipment required to obtain dynamic strength measurements and static strength measurements.

F. Describe five examples of exercise programs for participants identified as being deficient in flexibility of the following: hip, knee joint, trunk, shoulder.

G. Explain three techniques and procedures in the use of exercise test data for exercise prescription.

H. Outline two methods of designing exercise programs of a progressive intensity and two methods of determining optimum target exercise intensity.

I. Outline five specific physical activities designed to increase aerobic capacity with a group of men whose estimated aerobic capacity is 31.5 ml O_2/kg min.

J. Discuss each of the following topics for a period of ten minutes and support the presentation with published research evidence: diet and weight control; exercise and the heart; physical fitness programs; heart disease and risk factors; the role of training and conditioning on human performance and on anxiety, stress and relaxation in daily life.

K. Show the following methods of obtaining participant's heart rates during activity sessions (radial, brachial, carotid, subclavian, thoracic).

G.O. The exercise leader will demonstrate his understanding of therapeutic exercise and exercise prescription.

S.L.O. Given a number of patients with a variety of performance capabilities and medical problems, the exercise leader will:

A. Measure joint range of motion of the leg, spine, shoulder and forearm.

B. Use the goniometer and produce replicable measurements on five of the above patients.

C. Execute twenty warm-up exercises and discuss the purpose of each.

D. Lead an exercise session. The following characteristics must be shown for competency.

1. Rhythm (sequence or beat)
2. Timing
3. Intensity
4. Diversity of activity

6. *Exercise Laboratory Techniques*
   G.O. The exercise leader will understand exercise laboratory techniques.
   S.L.O. Refer to S.L.O.'s for exercise technician.

7. *Internship*

In order to qualify as an exercise leader, an internship of at least six months is necessary. This internship should occur under the direction of an established program director who is an active leader in physical activity programs of intervention and rehabilitation. The internship should consist of a wide variety of experiences to include: progressive exercise testing, exercise prescription and exercise session leadership. Evaluation of the exercise leader will involve the demonstration of proficiency in leading activity plus oral and written examinations in the above content areas (1 to 6).

EXERCISE TECHNICIAN

The major role of the exercise technician is to administer graded exercise tests safely and reproducibly so as to obtain reliable and valid data. Depending on the health status and age of the participant, the exercise technician may administer the test on his own initiative or under the direct supervision of a program director or a physician. Therefore, he must be able to judge appropriate initial levels of work for diverse populations based on history and physical examination. He must also be able to assess the increments in progressive work demands that are appropriate on the basis of the participants' response to the preceding workload.

The exercise technician must be able to communicate well with physicians, program directors, exercise leaders, subjects and patients. In addition to communicating well with test participants, he must develop rapport with them so that he has their trust and confidence.

Although the role of the exercise technician is the preparation for and the administration of the graded exercise test, his skills in working with individual subjects and patients during graded exercise will enable him to undertake other roles in exercise programs. When necessary, he could supervise prescribed exercise of individual subjects or patients under the direct supervision of a physician, program director or exercise leader.

The following professional training lends itself to future education and experience as an exercise technician: physical education, nursing, physical therapy, occupational therapy, laboratory technology and medical technology.

The role and responsibility of the exercise technician are as follows: to prepare the graded exercise station for administration of tests, screen patients for graded exercise testing, administer graded exercise test, calculate data obtained during graded exercise, implement emergency procedures and to interact and communicate with the physician, program director, exercise leader, subjects and patients.

The primary responsibility of the exercise technician is the administration of the graded exercise test. This does not preclude the addition of other responsibilities due to the specific requirements of a given program. Several items are listed as "optional." Optional items may or may not be included in graded exercise testing but it would be advantageous for exercise technicians to know such procedures.

1. *Mechanics of Individual Test Procedures*

   G.O. The exercise technician will understand the sterilization of equipment.

   S.L.O. Given a list representative of equipment used in progressive exercise testing, the exercise technician will:

   A. List three types of equipment that must be sterilized after each test and also the storage procedure for each.

   B. List five steps required to sterilize each piece of equipment.

   G.O. The exercise technician will demonstrate his understanding of the administration of standard 12 lead resting electrocardiogram (ECG).

   S.L.O. Given a subject who will undergo a progressive exercise test, the exercise technician will:

   A. Set up and calibrate the ECG recorder for a 10-mV pen deflection.

   B. Prepare three skin sites for electrode placement and describe their use.

   C. Place the electrodes at the appropriate sites listed above.

   D. Select the correct inputs to record each of the 12 leads.

   E. Obtain a readable tracing of each lead with standardization.

   F. Mount a representative tracing of each lead to include abnormalities for permanent record.

G. Clean up and store equipment. Make sure all paste is removed from the electrodes.

G.O. The exercise technician will demonstrate his understanding of the measurement of blood pressure.

S.L.O. Given a subject who will undergo a progressive exercise stress test, the exercise technician will:

A. List the five phases of sound as cuff pressure is reduced from above systolic to below diastolic pressures.

B. Apply blood pressure cuff securely to the arm in preparation for an exercise test.

C. With patient at rest, take systolic and diastolic blood pressure by the auscultatory method using first, fourth and fifth phase.

D. During graded exercise, take systolic and diastolic blood pressure by the auscultatory method using first, fourth and fifth phase.

G.O. The exercise technician will demonstrate his understanding of the measurement of ventilation (optional).

S.L.O. Given equipment which measures respiratory responses, the exercise technician will:

A. Set up the equipment for collection of expired gas by Douglas bag method.

B. List the steps required to measure minute ventilation ($\dot{V}E$), tidal volume (VT), respiratory rate (f) for the Douglas bag method.

C. Collect data necessary to measure $\dot{V}E$, VT and f at rest and during exercise.

    D. Calculate $\dot{V}E$ (liters/min), ATPS, BTPS and STPD; VT and f from the above data.

    E. List five steps in calibrating the dry gas meter.

    F. Set up equipment necessary for measurement of inspired gas volume by dry gas meter.

G.O. The exercise technician will apply the proper procedures in the measurement of O_2 intake (optional).

S.L.O. Given a micro-Scholander or Haldane Gas Analyzer, the exercise technician will:

    A. Set up gas analyzer and mix chemicals necessary for absorption within a 90-minute period of time.

    B. Insert gas sample and manipulate apparatus to obtain micrometer reading for carbon dioxide (CO_2) and oxygen (O_2).

    C. Calculate the percentage of CO_2 in sample and reproduce consecutive readings of the same gas sample to within a .05% error.

G.O. The exercise technician will demonstrate competency in the use of the electronic gas analyzer (optional).

S.L.O. Given an electronic analyzer, the exercise technician will:

    A. Set up and calibrate CO_2 and O_2 analyzer with three separate test gases.

    B. Sample the composition of a Douglas bag and obtain a read-out on recorder or instrument.

    C. Calculate percentage of CO_2 and O_2 in gas

sample and reproduce two consecutive readings within the accuracy of the instrument.

G.O. The exercise technician will demonstrate competency in collecting data necessary in evaluating metabolic response.

S.L.O. Given the necessary equipment and a subject to be evaluated, the exercise technician will:

A. List the measurements and factors necessary to calculate O_2 intake and CO_2 production.

B. Collect data necessary to calculate O_2 intake and CO_2 production and calculate O_2 intake, METS, CO_2 production and respiratory exchange ratio.

G.O. The exercise technician will demonstrate competence in the use of the ECG.

S.L.O. Given equipment and a variety of subjects, the exercise technician will:

A. Select the appropriate sites for placing chest electrodes, prepare the sites properly and place electrodes to obtain a readable ECG recording free of interference during exercise.

B. Set up and calibrate recorder and oscilloscope for the recording of the exercise ECG.

C. When presented with an ECG abnormality, identify and stop, if indicated, the exercise test.

G.O. The exercise technician will demonstrate the ability to select workloads in graded exercise.

S.L.O. Given body weight, the exercise technician will:
Manipulate step height and cadence on steps, load and pedaling speed on the

bicycle ergometer and grade and speed on treadmill to obtain given workloads in METS.

S.L.O. Given prescribed intensities for stepping, cycling or running work and the subject's weight, the exercise technician will:

Calculate the number of METS required to perform the activity.

S.L.O. Given data on or after screening a subject or patient, the exercise technician will:

Set appropriate initial work level on steps, bicycle ergometer or treadmill.

S.L.O. Given screening data and response to previous work level, the exercise technician will:

Set appropriate increment in work on steps, bicycle ergometer and treadmill.

G.O. The exercise technician will demonstrate competency in exercise stress tests.

S.L.O. Given three subjects and a series of protocols, the exercise technician will:

A. Administer a continuous and discontinuous test using a bicycle ergometer and a motor driven treadmill.

B. Stop test on the appearance of appropriate signs, symptoms or physiological responses (ECG, HR or blood pressure).

G.O. The exercise technician will understand emergency procedures in exercise stress tests (see Guidelines, p. 26).

S.L.O. Given ten possible emergencies during an exercise stress test, the exercise technician will:

List, describe and implement the appropriate emergency procedure for each given situation.

2. *Screening a Patient Before Exercise Testing*

G.O. The exercise technician will demonstrate competence in screening a patient before exercise testing.

S.L.O. Given a number of patients with a wide variety of medical problems requiring a progressive exercise test evaluation, the exercise technician will:

A. Question patient to obtain recent history relevant to: angina, shortness of breath and dyspnea, sleep, communicable diseases, drug usage and work capacity.

B. Take oral temperatures, compare them to normal values, and determine whether or not they are within the normal range.

C. Take resting blood pressures, compare to normal values, and determine whether or not they are within the normal range.

D. Take standard 12 lead ECG, for each of the given patients.

E. Administer the informed consent form to each of the subjects or patients.

F. Report items identified in the screening process which should require the physician's attention.

3. *Administration of Graded Exercise Test*

G.O. The exercise technician will demonstrate the ability to administer a graded exercise test.

S.L.O. Given a series of patients with a wide variety of performance capabilities, the exercise technician will:

    A. Select the initial workload, in consultation with the physician, based on the estimated performance capabilities of the patients.

    B. Accurately monitor the heart rate and ECG, obtain reliable blood pressures and when required, obtain accurate measurements of respiratory gas exchange.

    C. Stop exercise test when visual or physiological signs or symptoms suggest further exercise is contraindicated.

    D. Obtain a post exercise standard 12 lead ECG if it is part of the protocol.

4. *Post Exercise Procedures*

    G.O. The exercise technician will demonstrate his understanding of post exercise procedures.

    S.L.O. Given a series of patients who have completed a graded exercise test and the following recovery period, the exercise technician will:

        A. Remove electrodes, cuff and other test equipment and encourage the subject or patient to move around and cool down gradually.

        B. Direct each patient, after the cool-down period, to shower. Insist that shower door not be locked and that he/she continually moves the lower extremities.

    G.O. The exercise technician will demonstrate his

understanding of laboratory procedures and equipment used in a progressive exercise test.

S.L.O. Given a series of patients who have showered and are being prepared for discharge from the testing site, the exercise technician will:

A. Turn off or put recorders on stand-by and wash and sterilize equipment according to proper procedures.

B. Organize and calculate test data in a sequential manner, and present them to the physician or program director.

*Informed Consent for Graded Exercise Test**

1. *Explanation of the Graded Exercise Test*

   You will perform a graded exercise test on a bicycle ergometer and/or a motor-driven treadmill. The work levels will begin at a level you can easily accomplish and will be advanced in stages, depending on your work capacity. We may stop the test at any time because of signs of fatigue or you may stop when you wish to because of personal feelings of fatigue or discomfort. We do not wish you to exercise at a level which is abnormally uncomfortable for you.

2. *Risks and Discomforts*

   There exists the possibility of certain changes occurring during the test. They include abnormal blood pressure, fainting, disorders of heart beat, and very rare instances of heart attack. Every effort will be made to minimize them by the preliminary examination and by observations during testing. Emergency equipment and trained personnel are available to deal with unusual situations which may arise.

3. *Benefits to be Expected*

   The results obtained from the exercise test may assist

---

* Where test is for a purpose other than prescription, *e.g.* experimental interest, this should be indicated on the Informed Consent Form.

in the diagnosis of your illnesses or in evaluating what types of activities you might carry out with no or low hazards.

4. *Inquiries*

Any questions about the procedures used in the graded exercise test or in the estimation of functional capacity are welcome. If you have any doubts or questions, please ask us for further explanations.

5. *Freedom of Consent*

Permission for you to perform this graded exercise test is voluntary. You are free to deny consent if you so desire.

I have read this form and I understand the test procedures that I will perform and I consent to participate in this test.

_____

Signature of Patient

_____   _____

Date   Witness

Appendix B

Medical Referral Form for Participation in Graded Exercise Test and Exercise Program

Patient's Name _____ Date_____
                Last   First   Initial

Address _____ Age _____ Phone _____

I consider the above individual as:

___ Normal

___ Cardiac Patient

___ Prone to Coronary Heart Disease

___ Other (Explain)_____

Diagnostic Data Etiologic	Present Physical Activity	ECG	Rhythm
1. No heart disease	1. Very active	1. Normal	1. Sinus
2. Rheumatic heart disease	2. Normal	2. Dig. Effect Only	2. Atrial fib.
3. Congenital heart disease	3. Limited	3. Abnormal	3. Other
4. Hypertension	4. Very limited	4. Infarct	
5. Ischemic heart disease			
6. Other			

101

Specific Cardiac Diagnosis _____

_____

Additional Abnormalities you are aware of _____

_____

Date of Last Complete Physical Examination _____

Present Medication _____

Please fill in the information below if it is available:

1. Urine, sp.gr._____ Alb._____ Glucose_____ Micro._____

2. Complete blood count: Hbg.__ Hct.__ WBC__ Diff.__

3. ECG, 12 lead (enclose copy) _____

4. Blood pressure, syst.__diast.__

5. Glucose_____mg.%

6. 2 Hr. Post Dexicola_____mg.%

7. Cholesterol_____mg.% Lipoprotein Electrophoresis_____
   Triglyceride_____mg.%

8. Graded Exercise Test Results (If available, enclose)

Impression of above information _____

_____

The above listed person is capable of participating in an

exercise program as well as periodic laboratory evaluations, under the guidance and supervision of a

( ) Physician
( ) Exercise Leader (____) Check appropriate supervision (____).

Signed:_____M.D.

Type or Print
Name of Physician_____

Address _____ Telephone No._____

Appendix C

Medication Deletion Instructions
Before Diagnostic Exercise Stress Testing

Trade Name of Medication	Generic Name* of Medication	Purpose	Washout Time
Acetazolamide*	See DIAMOX		
ALDACTAZIDE	Spironolactone with hydrochlorothiazide	antihypertensive, diuretic	2–3 days
ALDACTONE	Spironolactone	antihypertensive, diuretic	2–3 days
ALDOMET	Methyldopa	antihypertensive	48 hours

Trade Name of Medication	Generic Name* of Medication	Purpose	Washout Time
ALDORIL	Methyldopa and hydrochlorothiazide	antihypertensive, diuretic	48 hours
Allopurinol*	See ZYLOPRIM		
Amitriptyline*	See ELAVIL		
APRESOLINE HYDROCHLORIDE	Hydralazine hydrochloride	antihypertensive	2 weeks
ATROMID S	Clofibrate	lipid lowering agent	Continue as usual
BENTYL	Dicyclomine hydrochloride N.F.	gastrointestinal antispasmodic	12 hours
BRONKOTABS	Ephedrine, etc.	bronchodilator	24 hours
CARDILATE	Erythrityl tetranitrate	coronary vasodilator, anti-anginal	24 hours
CARDIOQUIN	Quinidine polygalacturonate	antiarrhythmic agent	5 days
Chlordiazepoxide hydrochloride*	See LIBRIUM		

Chlorothiazide*	See DIURIL	
Chlorothiazide and Reserpine*	See DIUPRES	
Chlorpromazine*	See THORAZINE	
Chlorthalidone*	See HYGROTON	
Clofibrate*	See ATROMID S	
COUMADIN	Crystalline sodium warfarin	anticoagulant	Continue as usual
DIAMOX	Acetazolamide	diuretic	24 hours
Diazepam*	See VALIUM	
Dicyclomine hydrochloride N.F.*	See BENTYL	
Digitoxin Tablets U.S.P.*	—	digitalis preparation	2–3 weeks
Digoxin*	See LANOXIN	
DIUPRES	Chlorothiazide and Reserpine	antihypertensive, diuretic	1–2 weeks

Trade Name of Medication	Generic Name* of Medication	Purpose	Washout Time
DIURIL	Chlorothiazide	diuretic	24 hours
DYAZIDE	Dyrenium and hydrochlorothiazide	diuretic	48 hours
DYRENIUM	Triamterene	diuretic	48 hours
Dyrenium and hydro-chlorothiazide*	See DYAZIDE		
ELAVIL	Amitriptyline	antidepressant	14 days
ENDURON	Methyclothiazide	antihypertensive, diuretic	24 hours
Erythrityl tetranitrate*	See CARDILATE		
ESIDRIX	Hydrochlorothiazide	diuretic	24 hours
Furosemide*	See LASIX		
Guanethidine sulfate*	See ISMELIN		

108

Hydralazine hydrochloride*	See APRESOLINE HYDROCHLORIDE	
Hydrochlorothiazide*	See ESIDRIX, HYDRODIURIL	
HYDRODIURIL	Hydrochlorothiazide	antihypertensive, diuretic	6–12 hours
HYGROTON	Chlorthalidone	antihypertensive, diuretic	48–72 hours
Imipramine hydrochloride*	See TOFRANIL	
INDERAL	Propranolol hydrochloride	beta blocker, anti-anginal drug, anti-arrhythmic	1–2 weeks
ISMELIN	Guanethidine sulfate	antihypertensive	7–21 days
Isoproterenol hydrochloride*	See ISUPREL HYDROCHLORIDE	
ISORDIL	Isosorbide dinitrate	coronary vasodilator, anti-anginal	2–3 hours

Trade Name of Medication	Generic Name* of Medication	Purpose	Washout Time
ISORDIL TEMBIDS	Isosorbide dinitrate	long-acting coronary vasodilator, anti-anginal	8–10 hours
Isosorbide dinitrate*	See ISORDIL, ISORDIL TEMBIDS, SORBITRATE		
ISUPREL HYDROCHLORIDE	Isoproterenol hydrochloride	bronchodilator	4 hours
KAON	Potassium gluconate	oral potassium	1 week
LANOXIN	Digoxin	digitalis preparation	1 week
LASIX	Furosemide	antihypertensive, diuretic	24 hours
LIBRIUM	Chlordiazepoxide hydrochloride	tranquilizer	Continue as usual
MELLARIL	Thioridazine	tranquilizer	2–4 weeks
Meprobamate*	See MILTOWN		
Methyclothiazide*	See ENDURON		

Methyldopa*	See ALDOMET		
Methyldopa and hydrochlorothiazide*	See ALDORIL		
MILTOWN	Meprobamate	tranquilizer	Continue as usual
MYLANTA	Aluminum hydroxide, etc.	antacid	Continue as usual
NITROBID	Nitroglycerin	long-acting coronary vasodilator, anti-anginal	8–12 hours
Nitroglycerin*	—	coronary vasodilator, anti-anginal	2 hours
Nitroglycerin*	See NITROBID, NITROGLYN		
NITROGLYN	Nitroglycerin, glyceryl trinitrate	long-acting coronary vasodilator, anti-anginal	12 hours
PAPAVATRAL 20	Ethaverine, pentaerythritol tetranitrate	long-acting coronary vasodilator, anti-anginal	12 hours
Pentaerythritol tetranitrate*	See PERITRATE SA		

Trade Name of Medication	Generic Name* of Medication	Purpose	Washout Time
PERITRATE SA	Pentaerythritol tetranitrate	long-acting coronary vasodilator	24 hours
Potassium gluconate*	See KAON		
Procainamide hydrochloride	See PRONESTYL		
PRONESTYL	Procainamide hydrochloride	antiarrhythmic	1 week
Propranolol hydrochloride*	See INDERAL		
QUADRINAL	Ephedrine, phenobarb, theophylline, iodide	bronchodilator	24 hours
QUINAGLUTE DURA-TABS	Quinidine gluconate	antiarrhythmic	5 days
Quinidine gluconate	See QUINAGLUTE DURA-TABS		
Quinidine polygalacturonate*	See CARDIOQUIN		

Quinidine Sulfate*	—	antiarrhythmic	5 days
RAUDIXIN	Rauwolfia serpentina	antihypertensive	2 weeks
Rauwolfia serpentina*	See RAUDIXIN		
REGROTON	Chlorthalidone and reserpine	antihypertensive	2 weeks
Reserpine*	See SERPASIL, REGROTON		
SERPASIL	Reserpine	antihypertensive	2 weeks
SORBITRATE	Isosorbide dinitrate	coronary vasodilator, anti-anginal	4 hours
Spironolactone*	See ALDACTONE		
Spironolactone with hydrochlorothiazide*	See ALDACTAZIDE		
STELAZINE	Trifluoperazine hydrochloride	tranquilizer	1 week
TEDRAL	Theophylline, etc.	bronchodilator	24 hours
Thioridazine*	See MELLARIL		

Trade Name of Medication	Generic Name* of Medication	Purpose	Washout Time
THORAZINE	Chlorpromazine	tranquilizer	48 hours
TOFRANIL	Imipramine hydrochloride	antidepressant	48 hours
Triamterene*	See DYRENIUM		
Trifluoperazine hydrochloride*	See STELAZINE		
VALIUM	Diazepam	tranquilizer	Continue as usual
VEREQUAD	Ephedrine, theophylline, phenobarb	bronchodilator	24 hours
Warfarin*	See COUMADIN		
ZYLOPRIM	Allopurinol	antigout preparation	Continue as usual

Note: This listing was compiled from pharmaceutical company information modified according to clinical experience. It is recognized that at times blood level information conflicts with clinical evidence of continued biological activity of a preparation. When this occurred, the clinical impression of washout time has been listed. In no case should a drug be discontinued without the explicit consent of the family physician.

Appendix D
Informed Consent for
Outpatient Rehabilitation Program

1. *Explanation of Outpatient Rehabilitation Program*

    You will be placed on a rehabilitation program that will include physical exercises. The levels of exercise which you will undertake will be based on your cardiovascular response to an initial graded exercise test. You will be given explicit instructions regarding the amount and kind of daily exercise you should do. You will return once weekly as an outpatient for a rehabilitation session. This session is being held to evaluate your progress and to prescribe your daily exercise program for the subsequent week based on ECG and heart rate response to exercise. You will be given the opportunity for retests with the graded exercise test 3, 6, and 9 months after the initiation of the rehabilitation program.

2. *Telemetry*

    We will monitor your ECG during exercise. This will involve two or more electrodes being attached to your chest and perhaps carrying a small transmitter. The ECG signal will be picked up by a receiver.

3. *Risks and Discomforts*

    There exists the possibility of certain changes occurring during the tests. They include abnormal blood pressure, fainting, disorders of heart beat, and very rare instances of heart attack. Every effort will be made to minimize them by the preliminary examination and by observations during testing. Emergency equipment and trained personnel are available to deal with unusual situations which may arise.

4. *Benefits to be Expected*

Participation in the rehabilitation program may not benefit you directly in any way. The results obtained may help in evaluating what type of activities you might carry out safely in your daily life. No assurance can be given that the rehabilitation program will increase your functional capacity although widespread experience indicates that improvement is usually achieved.

5. *Inquiries*

Any questions about the rehabilitation program are welcome. If you have doubts or questions, please ask us for further explanation.

6. *Freedom of Consent*

Permission for you to engage in this Rehabilitation Program is voluntary. You are free to deny consent if you so desire, both now and at any point in the program.

I have read this form and understand the Rehabilitation Program in which I will be engaged. I consent to participate in this Rehabilitation Program.

_____

Signature of Patient

_____   _____

Date   Witness